Biomaterials

Edited by Petrică Vizureanu
and Claudia Manuela Da Cunha Ferreira Botelho

Published in London, United Kingdom

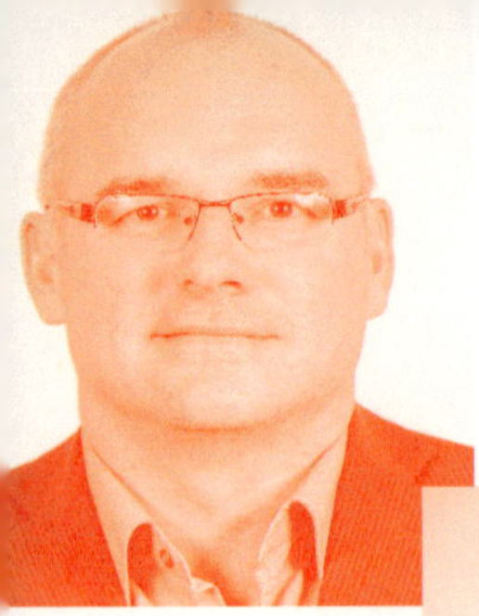
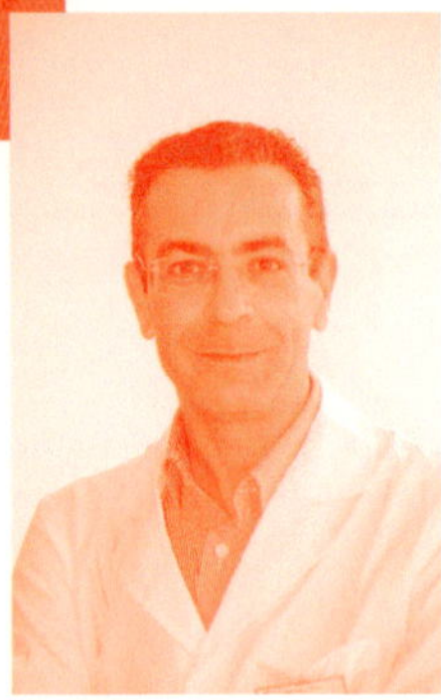
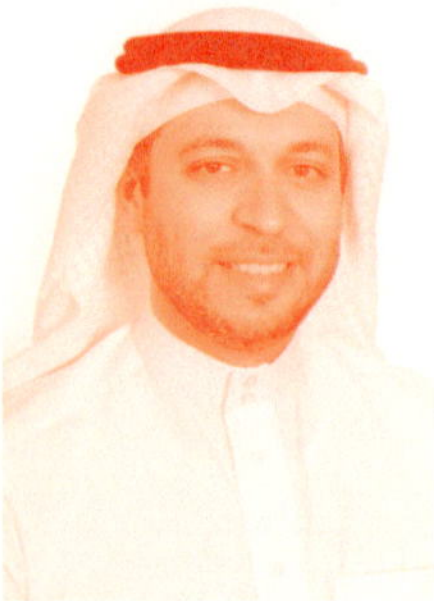
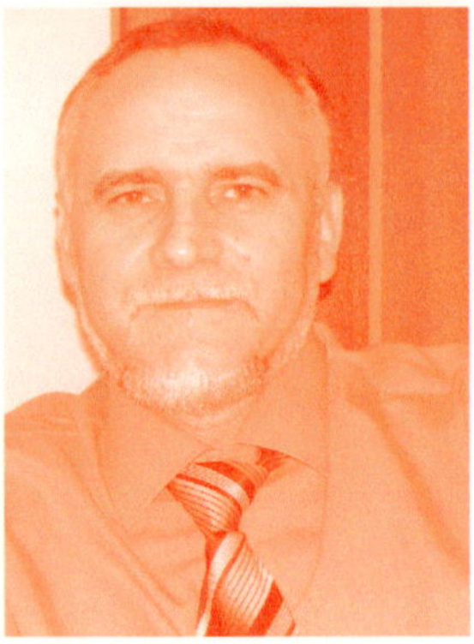
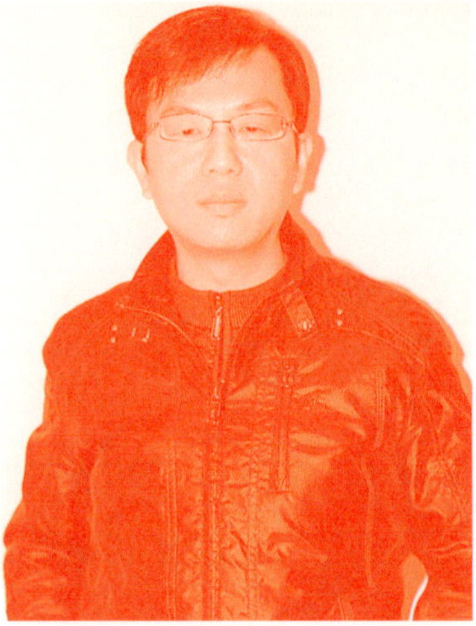
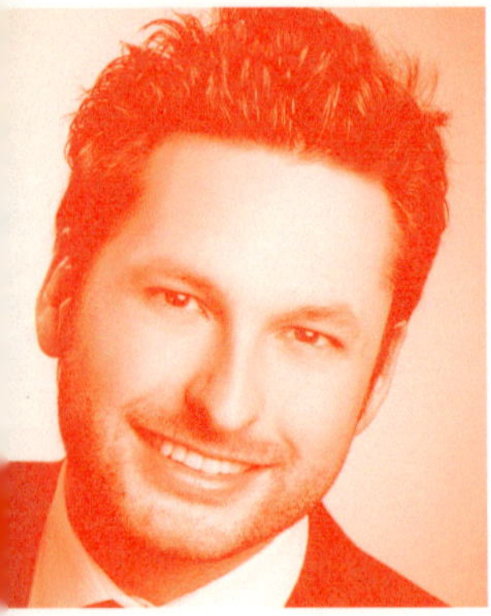
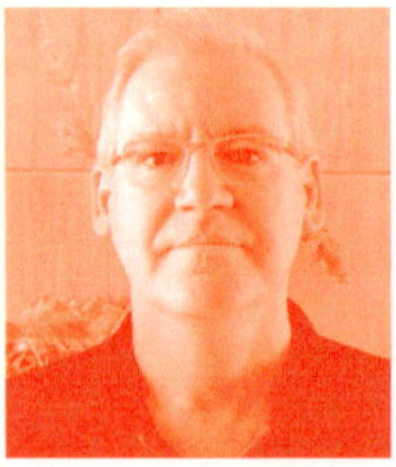

IntechOpen

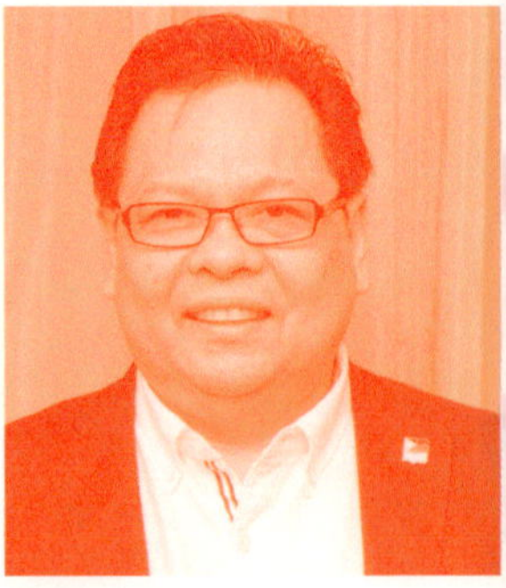
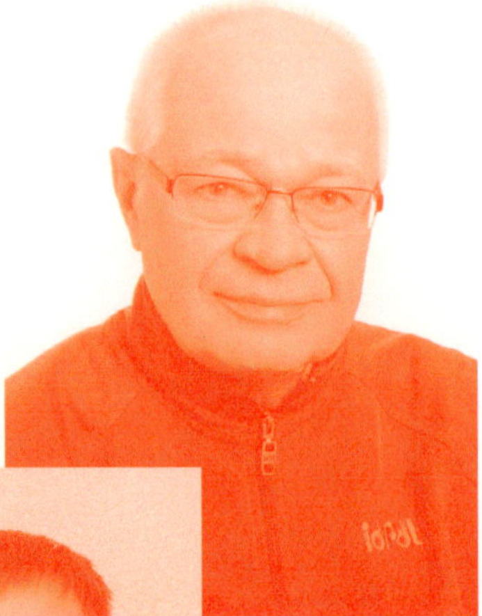
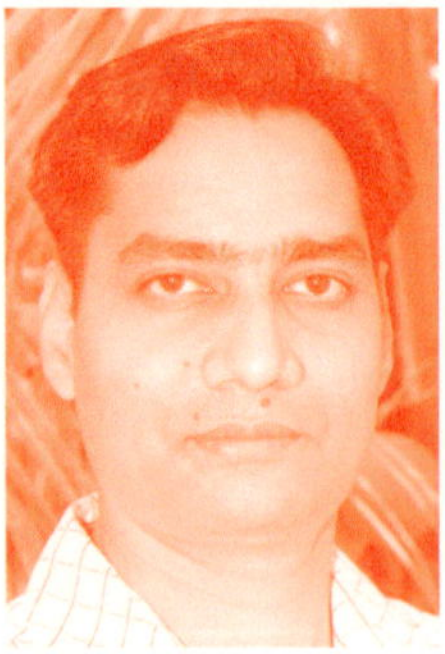
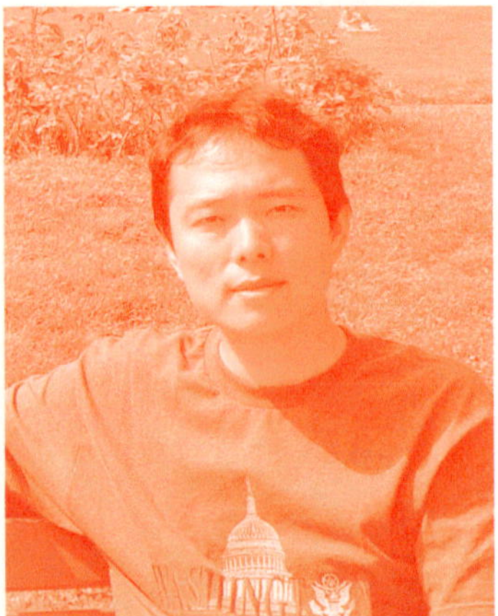
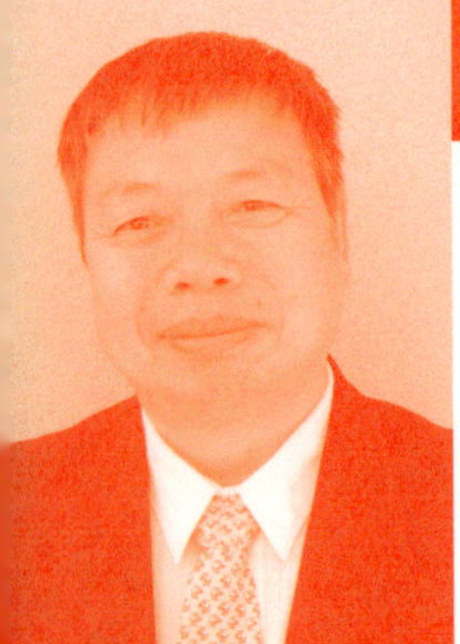
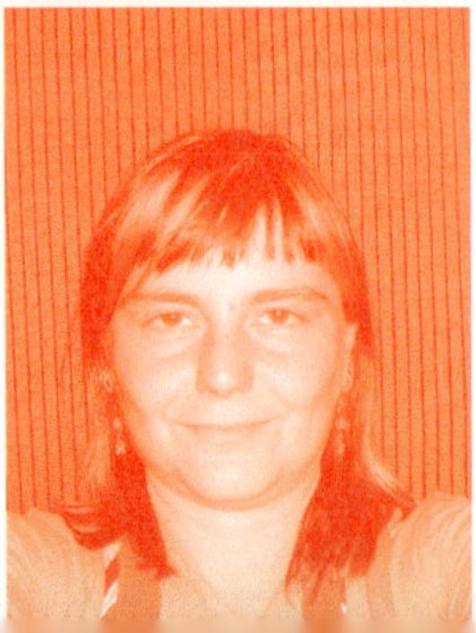

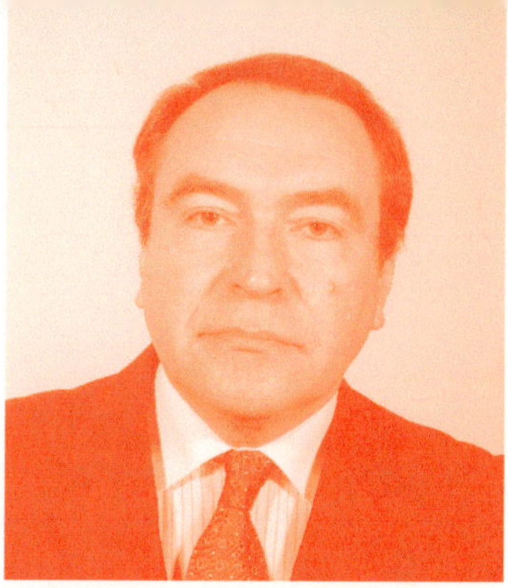
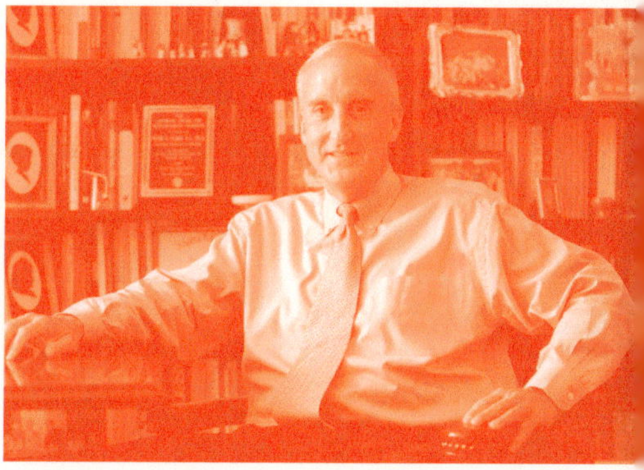
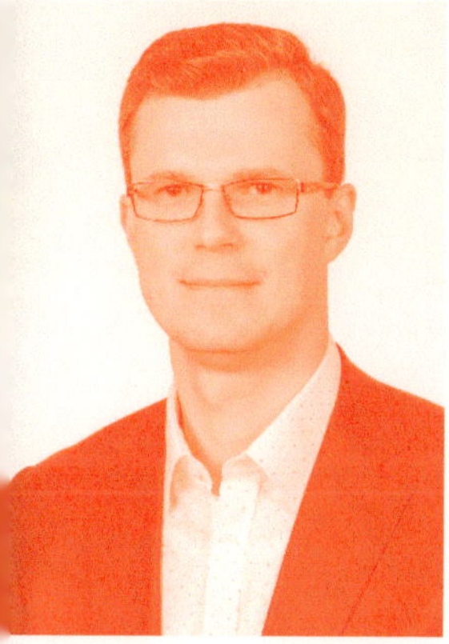
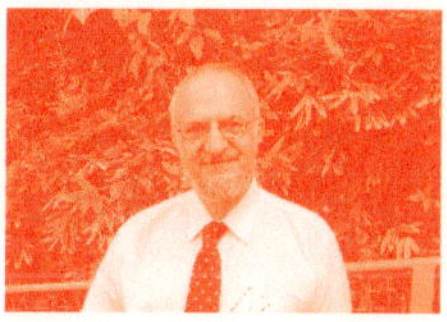
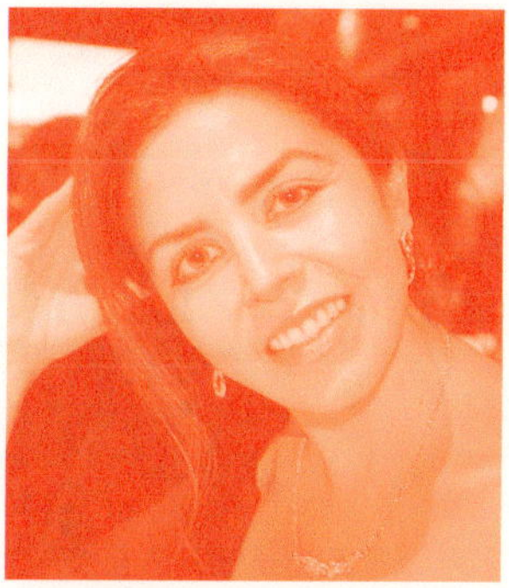

Supporting open minds since 2005

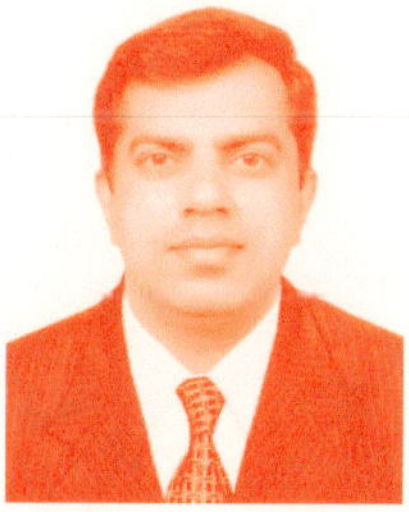
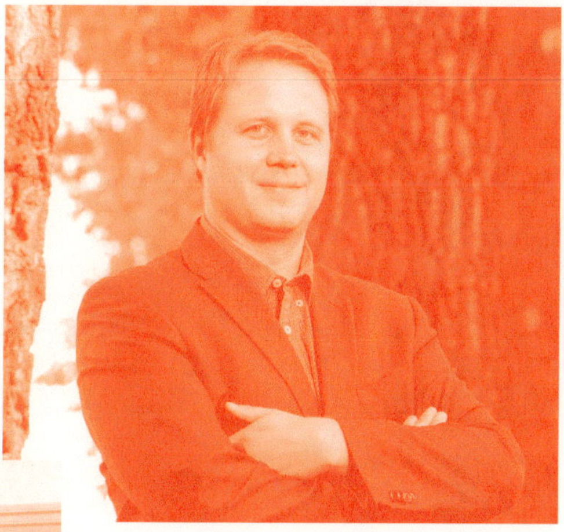
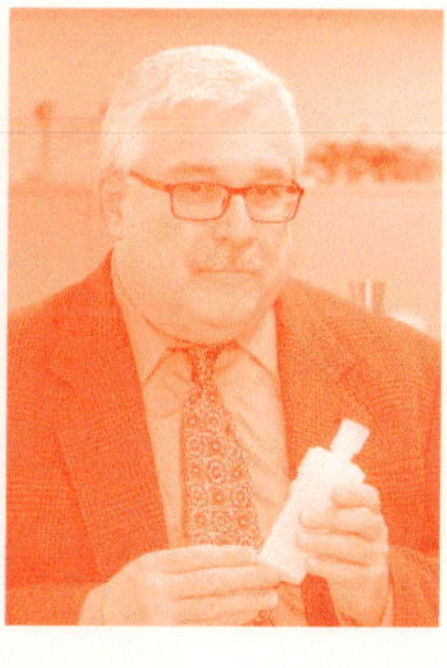
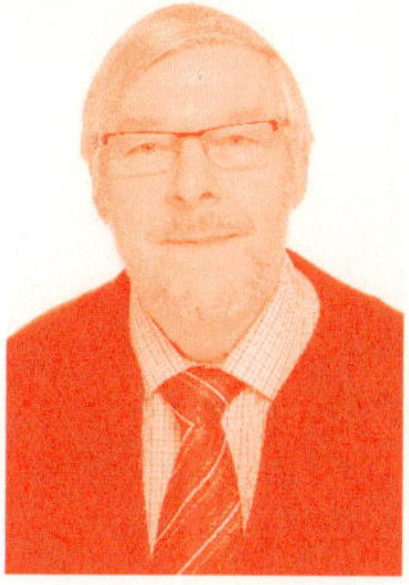
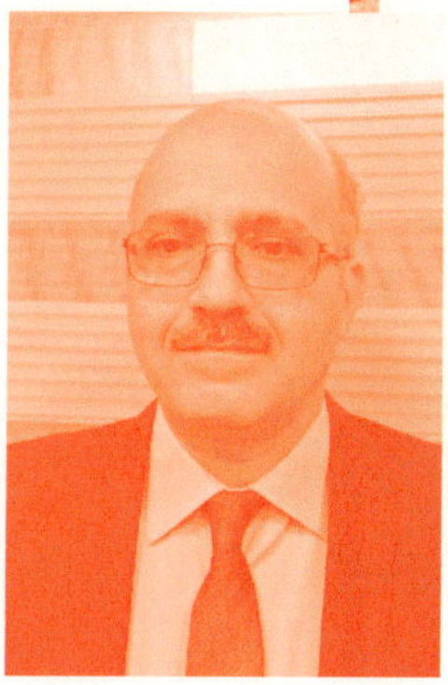
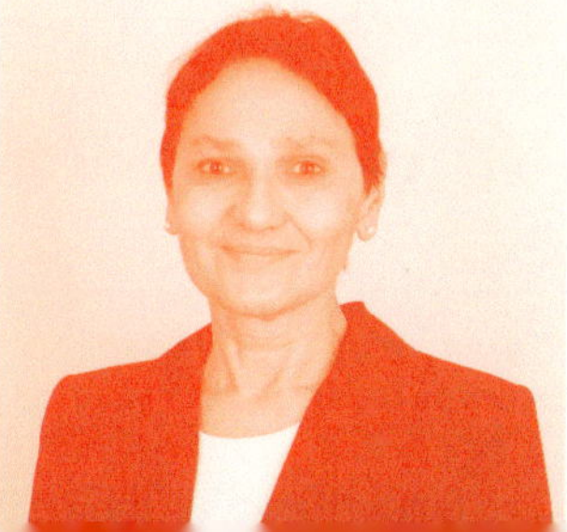
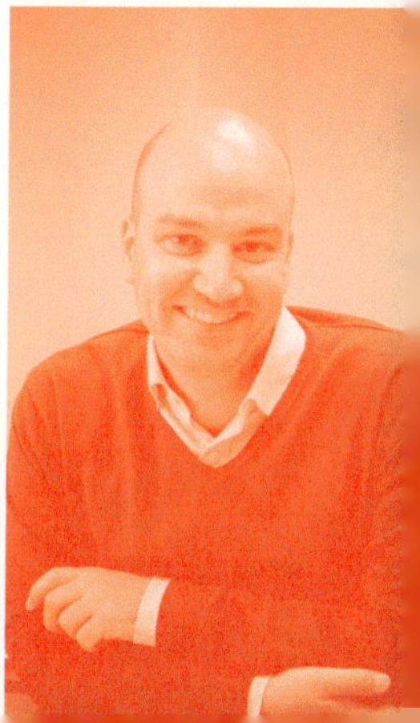

Biomaterials
http://dx.doi.org/10.5772/intechopen.87369
Edited by Petrică Vizureanu and Claudia Manuela Da Cunha Ferreira Botelho

Contributors
Bernard O. Asimeng, Elvis Kwason Tiburu, David W. Afeke, Md. Shariful Islam, Md. Abdulla-Al-Mamun, Alam Khan, Mitsugu Todo, Yvonne Reinwald, Roxana Mioara Piticescu, Laura Madalina Cursaru, Gabriela Negroiu, Cristina Florentina Ciobota, Ciprian Neagoe, Daniel Safranchik, Petrică Vizureanu, Madalina Simona Baltatu, Andrei Victor Sandu, Alper Gultekin, Caglar Cinar, Alper Saglanmak, Cem Töre, Narayana Kalkura, Andrea Domingues Goncalves, Wendy Balestri, Kumaravelu Thanigai Arul, Jayapalan Ramana Ramya

First published in London, United Kingdom, 2020 by IntechOpen
IntechOpen is the global imprint of INTECHOPEN LIMITED, registered in England and Wales, registration number: 11086078, 5 Princes Gate Court, London, SW7 2QJ, United Kingdom
Printed in Croatia

British Library Cataloguing-in-Publication Data
A catalogue record for this book is available from the British Library

Additional hard and PDF copies can be obtained from orders@intechopen.com

Biomaterials
Edited by Petrică Vizureanu and Claudia Manuela Da Cunha Ferreira Botelho
p. cm.
Print ISBN 978-1-78984-464-1
Online ISBN 978-1-78984-465-8
eBook (PDF) ISBN 978-1-83962-739-2

For EU product safety concerns:
IN TECH d.o.o., Prolaz Marije Krucifikse Kozulić 3, 51000 Rijeka, Croatia, info@intechopen.com or visit our website at intechopen.com.

Meet the editors

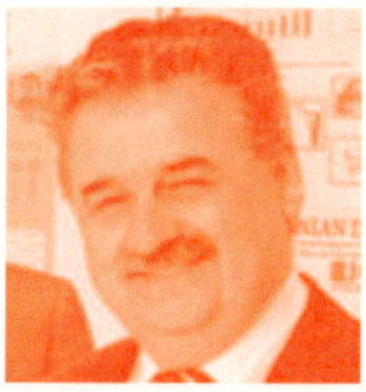

Petrică Vizureanu was born on October 17, 1967, in Bârlad, Romania. He obtained an MSc and PhD in Heating Equipment from The "Gheorghe Asachi" Technical University, Iasi, Romania in 1992 and 1999, respectively. Dr. Vizureanu is currently full Professor and Scientific Supervisor in Materials Engineering (since 2009) at the same university. His research focuses on expert systems for heating system programming, computer-assisted design for heating equipment, heating equipment for materials processing, heat transfer, biomaterials, and geopolymers. He has published more than 140 papers in international journals and conference proceedings, and thirty-three books.

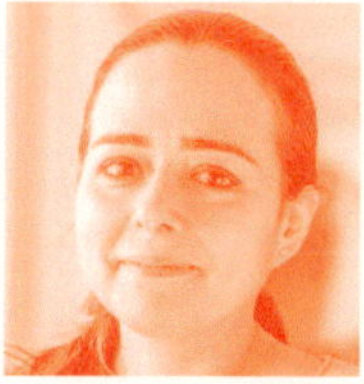

Claudia Botelho obtained a PhD in Science Engineering from Porto University, Portugal, in 2005. From 2001 to 2006 her research was carried out in the United Kingdom and Japan, where she focused on the development of custom-made ceramic prostheses for reconstructive surgery. In 2013 she was invited as a lecturer at Minho University, Portugal. Her work was distinguished with several international prizes, like the European Award on Biomaterials and Tissue Engineering Doctoral Award. Dr. Botelho has supervised many graduate and postgraduate theses. In 2015 she was elected president of the National Researcher Association of Science and Technology, collaborating development of new scientific policies. Currently, she is focusing on the characterisation of natural molecules that can be encapsulated into new developed cubosomes.

Contents

Preface

Globally, there is a continuous concern for research and development of alloys for medical and biomedical applications. The goal is to improve both the classic technologies of implant implementation and the technologies of synthesis of the biomaterials from which they are executed, with a final aim to promote a new generation of multifunctional implants with long-term performances.

Biomaterials have been used for several thousand years by ancient cultures in Egypt, Babylon, Greece, Italy, China, and Central and South America to replace different parts of the human bone system. These materials were used and developed before coining of the modern term "biompatibility," which was introduced about 60 years ago when researchers began to study and develop this field.

Biomaterials must be **biocompatible**, meaning they must be non-toxic and not release ions so that they can be tolerated by the human body for long periods of time (decades). They must also have certain **mechanical properties**, including mechanical stability depending on the application in which they are used, and they must resist demands and not break or deform excessively over time. Finally, biomaterials require **efficiency**, that is, they must be reliable, accessible, cost-effective, easy to process, and sterile. Considering all this, when obtaining biomaterials, raw materials of high purity are selected and the influence of the alloying elements must be studied.

The global biomaterials market is constantly growing due to an increasing population that is susceptible to diseases, such as cardiovascular, dental, orthopedic, and neurological conditions. Expansion and improvement of the market are necessary to improve the health of patients and extend the duration of use of biomaterials in the human body.

This book provides an overview of biomaterials science with a focus on health and medical applications that can be improved with new biomaterials with non-allergenic elements. These materials are designed to meet functional requirements and overcome the disadvantages of classical alloys used as biomaterials in human tissue.

Over seven chapters, this volume explains the problems created by classical alloys and examines how the new generation of biomaterials helps both doctors and patients. What is remarkable for the domain of biomaterials is the evolution and substantial efforts that have been made every day for constant improvement.

This book is designed for students, doctors, patients, and researchers worldwide.

Petrică Vizureanu (Academic editor)
Gheorghe Asachi Technical University of Iași,
Romania

Claudia Manuela da Cunha Ferreira Botelho (Co-editor)
University of Minho,
Portugal

Section 1

Medical Devices

Chapter 1

Biomedical Implants for Regenerative Therapies

Andrea Domingues Goncalves, Wendy Balestri and Yvonne Reinwald

Abstract

Regenerative therapies aim to develop novel treatments to restore tissue function. Several strategies have been investigated including the use of biomedical implants as three-dimensional artificial matrices to fill the defect side, to replace damaged tissues or for drug delivery. Bioactive implants are used to provide growth environments for tissue formation for a variety of applications including nerve, lung, skin and orthopaedic tissues. Implants can either be biodegradable or non-degradable, should be nontoxic and biocompatible, and should not trigger an immunological response. Implants can be designed to provide suitable surface area-to-volume ratios, ranges of porosities, pore interconnectivities and adequate mechanical strengths. Due to their broad range of properties, numerous biomaterials have been used for implant manufacture. To enhance an implant's bioactivity, materials can be functionalised in several ways, including surface modification using proteins, incorporation of bioactive drugs, growth factors and/or cells. These strategies have been employed to create local bioactive microenvironments to direct cellular responses and to promote tissue regeneration and controlled drug release. This chapter provides an overview of current bioactive biomedical implants, their fabrication and applications, as well as implant materials used in drug delivery and tissue regeneration. Additionally, cell- and drug-based bioactivity, manufacturing considerations and future trends will be discussed.

Keywords: biomaterials, bioactive biomedical implants, stem cells, drug delivery, manufacturing

1. Introduction to bioactive implants

Implants are man-made devices that are fabricated for the implantation inside body to replace or support a biological structure, together with delivering drugs and monitoring body functions. They can remain in the body temporarily or permanently [1]. To date, biomedical implants are used not only as sensory devices [2]; brain and neural devices including neuronal, cochlear and retinal implants [3, 4]; subcutaneous implants [5]; cardiovascular devices such as vascular grafts, stent, heart valves, pacemakers [3]; sutures and wound dressings [6]; spinal [7] and dental implants [8]; cosmetic [9] and structural implants [10] including rods, braces, craniofacial, hip and knee replacements; but also as ophthalmic devices including glasses and contact lenses as well as insulin delivery devices [6].

IntechOpen

In recent years, scaffolds made of synthetic or natural polymers were developed to regenerate damaged or deteriorated tissues, or to deliver drugs to specific locations. Scaffolds are three-dimensional (3D) structures that mimic the native extracellular matrix (ECM) of tissues and provide a substrate for cell adhesion and proliferation.

These biomedical implants can be made of bioactive materials. The term "bioactive" means that a material can affect its surrounding tissue biologically. Scaffolds can include molecules that promote a biological response in the region where they are implanted. Moreover, cells can be included in these scaffolds to promote healing and regeneration, as they naturally secrete growth factors and cytokines [11].

The risks related to the surgery during the placement or removal of the implant include infection and implant failure. Also, inflammation reaction against the material or rejection needs to be taken into consideration [1]. Here, we report what it is known about bioactive biomedical implants, their desired properties and their applications, focusing on the techniques and materials used for their fabrication. We further provide an overview of cell-based and drug-based implants, implant manufacture and its considerations.

2. Biomaterials for implants in drug delivery and regenerative therapies

To assist native tissue regeneration or/and replacement, implants are made of biomaterials, which support cell and tissue growth through cell adhesion, proliferation and differentiation, prevent unwanted cell and tissue growth, tailor tissue response and prevent immunological responses [12].

Biomaterials have been used for controlled drug delivery systems, sutures and adhesives including biodegradable and non-biodegradable materials, cardiovascular grafts, reconstructive and orthopaedic implants, ophthalmic devices such as corneas and contact lenses, and dental implants [13]. Various types of materials have been used to produce biomedical implants. These include bioceramics, polymers, metals and composites, which are further discussed below. **Table 1** summarises current biomedical applications for biomaterials.

Application	Material	References
Ophthalmic applications (contact lenses, intraocular lenses)	Silicones, hydrogels	[14]
Cardiovascular applications (vascular prostheses, artificial valves, stents, cardiac-assisted pumps, blood bags and catheters)	Polymers, metals and ceramics; polyurethane (PU); polyesters (PE); polybutesters (PBE); polypropylene (PP) and PTFE; stainless steel	[15–21]
Central nervous system and peripheral nervous system (scaffolds for nerve regeneration)	Polycaprolactone (PCL), silk, collagen	[11, 22–26]
Orthopaedic applications (total hip replacement, hip arthroplasty, total knee arthroplasty, bone screws, orthodontic brackets and wires; bone fillers and scaffolds as bone replacements)	Chromium, cobalt, molybdenum, nickel, titanium and zirconium alloys, ultrahigh molecular weight polyethylene (UHMWPE), Ti-6Al-4V, ceramic-coated steels, stainless steel, copper; natural polymers like collagen, chitosan, alginates, synthetic polymers, ceramics like bioglasses, hydroxyapatite and beta-TCP; poly(L-lactic acid) (PLLA); poly(lactic acid), poly(lactic-co-glycolic acid) (PLGA), polycaprolactone (PCL)	[11, 12, 14, 27–33]

Table 1.
Examples of biomedical applications for currently used biomaterials.

2.1 Bioceramics

Ceramics are chemically inert and possess low thermal and electric conductivity as well as physical properties, which make them a suitable material glass for biomedical implants [34, 35]. Bioceramics are osteoinductive and osteoconductive and possess mechanical properties like native bone. Their use as biomedical implants prevents the transmission of diseases and immunogenicity. To date, bioceramics are utilised for dental, periodontal, maxillofacial and orthopaedic applications [36]. In comparison to non-resorbable bioceramics, degradable ceramics exhibit lower mechanical strength. Their chemical and physical composition determines their biological response [37].

Ceramics produced from aluminium, zirconium and titanium oxides possess bending, tensile and compressive strength at least 3 times higher than natural bone and are used mainly for pin-type dental implants and root- and endosteal plate forms [38]. The first zirconia implants were reported in the 1970s. These implants exhibited the ability to integrate into bone tissue, accumulate less plaque and provide improved aesthetics compared to titanium implants [39, 40]. Hence, titanium-zirconium alloys, also called Straumann Roxolid or Roxolit (TiZr1317), are often used as dental implants due to their enhanced mechanical properties and osseointegrative properties that are often used as dental implants [41].

Calcium phosphate-based bioceramics such as tricalcium phosphate (TCP) are similar in chemical composition to the inorganic phase natural bone tissue. TCP exhibits better biodegradation, restorability and bioactivity *in vivo* than hydroxyapatite and is commonly used for orthopaedic, dental and maxillofacial applications. Complete resorption of orthopaedic implants fabricated from TCP was reported after up to 2 years in the rat tibia and for the formation of cancellous bone [42].

Amorphous or low crystalline hydroxyapatite (HAp) is bioactive and bioresorbable. The preparation of synthetic HA at high temperatures results in high crystallinity. Biodegradation and resorbability of HAp are very slow. HAp bioceramics are commonly used for small defects in the case of bone loss or fractures of the tibia, calcaneus and vertebra. HAp is not employed for load-bearing bone applications because of its poor mechanical properties. The modification of HAp with strontium, magnesium and silicon ions resulted in enhanced mechanical and biological properties [43]. Improved bioresorbability was achieved by zinc—[44] and manganese—[45] substitution of HAp.

Dicalcium phosphates (DCP) are biodegradable ceramics composed of calcium phosphates and water. DCPs are widely added to material compositions to modify their physical properties. Dehydrated DCP is known as brushite, which is used in tibial plate and distal metaphysis bone fractures [46].

Historically, ceramics have been used as dental and orthopaedic implant materials. However, compared to other material classes, ceramics have not been used extensively as implant materials due to their limited load-bearing capacity [14].

2.2 Polymers

Polymers are macromolecules that consist of covalently bonded repeating units, which can be of the same (homopolymers) or different (co-polymers) molecule type [27]. A variety of natural and synthetic polymers are used as soft tissue transplants, facial prostheses, denture, hip and joint replacements as well as medical adhesives, sealants and coatings [14].

Polymers are commonly selected based on their physical characteristics, composition, and mechanical properties; how easily they can be modified and moulded; their heat and electric conductivity as well as their ability to integrate into and attach to native tissue [47].

2.2.1 Natural polymers

Natural polymers possess similar properties to native tissues. They are non-toxic and exhibit protein binding-sites and biochemical moieties that are important for tissue regeneration. However, natural polymers are often associated with immunological reactions, low mechanical strength and degradation at body temperature limiting their usability [14].

One of the most commonly used natural polymers is collagen. More than twenty different collagens are known in connective tissues such as bone, tendon, skin, cartilage and ligaments of the ECM of different species. Collagen type I is the main component in bone, skin and tendon, whereas type II is found in articular cartilage. Because of its abundance in nature, its importance for tissue homeostasis and growth, collagen has been investigated as material for bone, cartilage, tendon, skin and blood vessel regeneration [11]. In the clinic, collagen is used for the generation of dermal tissue, neo-tissue formation and wound healing [14]. Further natural polymers are chitosan, hyaluronic acid, fibrin and silk.

Silk, or silk fibroin, is a naturally occurring polymeric protein produced by insects and worms. The protein content gives rise to silk's biocompatibility and its high tensile strength making it an ideal biomaterial for biomedical applications as gels, sponges and films [11, 48–53]. Silk composites fabricated from silk-chitosan and silk-hydroxyapatite have been used to improve silk's elasticity, degradation and porosity [54, 55].

Hyaluronic acid (HA), a non-adhesive glycosaminoglycan (GAG), occurs mostly in connective, epithelial, and neural tissue [56]. HA is commonly used as hydrogel for the regeneration of bone, cartilage and the vascular system and for drug delivery [11].

Chitosan is a biodegradable polysaccharide produced through partial deacetylation of chitin. Chitosan scaffolds exhibit similar properties to naturally occurring GAGs, leading to their bioactivity, and support cellular adhesion [11, 57]. It has been investigated as scaffold material in combination with collagen and HA, as well as PCL for bone, cartilage and nerve regeneration [11].

2.2.2 Synthetic polymers

Synthetic polymers were developed with tailored physical and chemical properties depending on the desired application to overcome limitations of natural polymers. Synthetic polymers are linear, branched or cross-linked depending on their molecular arrangement [58] and possess amorphous or crystalline structures [27]. In addition, synthetic polymers are cheaper in production and enable improved functionality [11]. Commonly used synthetic polymers are poly(lactic acid-co-glycolic acid) (PLGA), polyglycolic acid (PGA), polylactic acid (PLA), polycaprolactone (PCL) and poly-hydroxybutyrate (PHB) [11, 27, 59, 60].

PGA, PLA and PCL are used for sutures, interference screws, fixation plates for meniscal repair and craniomaxillofacial fixtures and 3D scaffolds. However, they are known to induce inflammatory responses and are limited in mechanical integrity and controlled degradation. Hence, metal/polymer composites such as Mg/PCL have been developed [27]. Biodegradable synthetic polymers

Synthetic polymer	Application	References
Poly(L-lactic acid) (PLLA); poly (D-lactic acid) (PDLA)	Sutures, drug delivery, vascular grafts, bone screws, fixation pins, dermal filler for facial atrophy (Scultra™)	[11, 61]
Poly(lactic-co-glycolic acid) (PLGA)	Drug delivery	[11, 62]
Polycaprolactone (PCL)	Long-term implant, maxillo-cranial facial implant; drug release	[11, 63]
PCL-gelatin, PCL-chitosan, PCL-collagen	Tissue regeneration	[60, 64, 65]
Poly-para-dioxanone (PPD)	Internal fracture fixation, medical implant as films, foams and moulded scaffolds	[47, 66, 67]
Low-density polyethylene (LDPE), high-density polyethylene (HDPE)	Total hip arthroplasty and treatment of osteolysis as polymer-ceramic composites; rhinoplasty surgery	[68–71]
Poly(methyl methacrylate) (PMMA)	Orbital medical implants, rhinoplasty, cranioplasty, bone cement in hip joint replacement, dental implant for restoration and aesthetics	[72–76]
Polydimethylsiloxane (PDMS)	Enclosing implantable electronic devices and sensors, medical implants, oesophagus substitutes, catheters, shunts, blood pumps and peacemakers	[77–80]
Polyamides (PA), e.g., nylon and nylon-composites	Sutures, fabrication of dentures; scaffold materials and nanofillers for bone regeneration	[81, 82]
Carbon nanotubes (CNT) and composites	Metal coatings for load-bearing musculoskeletal implants to improve surface porosity, reduce metal ionisation and promote the formation of hydroxyapatite	[83]

Table 2.
Synthetic polymers commonly used for the fabrication of biomedical implants.

are chosen based on the required physical, chemical and mechanical material characteristics (**Table 2**).

2.3 Metals and alloys

Due to their mechanical properties, the ease of their processing and the possibility to sterilise them, metals and alloys are ideal materials for biomedical implants [34].

Metals are commonly used as load-bearing orthopaedic implants such as wires, screws, fixation plates, artificial joints for hips, knees, shoulders and ankles, as well as for dental, cardiovascular and craniofacial applications [14].

Novel magnesium alloys have been investigated for orthopaedic and cardiovascular applications [84, 85]. Combining magnesium alloys with aluminium or rare earth metals improves their mechanical properties [86, 87]. However, the accumulation of these elements is associated with neurotoxicity and hepatotoxicity [88]; hence, these alloys are not suitable for biomedical applications. Instead, extensive research is carried out to develop nontoxic magnesium alloys [89], such as Mg-Si and Mg-Sr alloys [90].

Titanium alloys are among the most commonly used metal alloys [91] due to their biocompatibility [92] and corrosion resistance [93]. Their composition and microstructure vary depending on their elemental composition [94]. The mechanical properties of B-titanium alloys have a Young's modulus like bone but possess a low fatigue strength. Their mechanical properties can be enhanced through the addition of silicon dioxide, zirconium dioxide and Yttrium oxide. Furthermore, to increase their wear resistance, titanium alloys are surface treated. Pure titanium alloys are used in pacemaker cases, ventricular devices, implantable drug pumps, screws and staples in spinal surgery, dental implants and craniofacial implants. Ti-6Al-4V alloys are used in hip and knee replacements and dental implants. Due to the release of aluminium and vanadium ions, which can cause neurological conditions such as Alzheimer's, Ti-6Al-4V alloys are not considered safe for long-term use. β-Titanium alloys substituted with stabilising elements like zirconium, tantalum and molybdenum are safer compared to Ti-6Al-4V [27], and alternative titanium alloys, vanadium free Ti-6Al-7Nb and Ti-5Al-2.5Fe, are being developed [95].

Titanium has become the material of choice for implants; however, components of prosthetics are still manufactured from gold alloys, stainless steel, nickel-chromium alloys and cobalt-chromium alloys [35]. Cobalt chromium alloys enable the fabrication of customised grafts including subperiosteal implants. They are mainly composed of cobalt, chromium and molybdenum, which give rise to corrosion resistance and mechanical properties [96, 97]. Stainless steel alloys such as iron-chromium-nickel-based alloys are used as orthopaedic implants such as ramus blade, ramus frame, stabiliser pins and some mucosal inserts. Due to its nickel content, these alloys possess a low corrosion resistance and induce immunological reactions in patients with nickel allergies [34, 38].

3. Implant properties

Implant materials should possess adequate chemical and physical properties to allow for host tissue infiltration and nutrient transport; biocompatibility to avoid immunological responses; and corrosion resistance, degradation and bioresorbability to enable normal cellular activity and controlled implant degradation [14, 27, 98]. In addition, temporary implants should possess a highly interconnected porous structure to allow cell migration and nutrient and waste transport, provide suitable surface topography to support cell adhesion and growth, as well as allow for the release of bioactive molecules if applicable [5, 11, 12].

Mechanical properties like Young's Modulus, tensile, compressive and shear strength, yield strength and fatigue strength are required to ensure uniform stress distribution, to minimise the movement or fracture of the implant [34].

3.1 Surface properties

Surface properties influence cell adhesion and cellular and tissue responses. Surface tension determines the wettability by a wetting fluid, such as blood or water [11, 34]. Implant surfaces are also categorised by roughness, texture and the orientation of irregularities [38, 99]. The surface textures can vary from concave or convex. Concave surface textures occur due to additive treatments such as hydroxyapatite coatings, whereas convex surfaces are created through etching and blasting. Furthermore, implant surfaces can either be isotropic, meaning that implant properties are independent from the measurement direction, or anisotropic, which means properties are directionally dependent [12, 34].

3.2 Corrosion and degradation of implants

3.2.1 Metal corrosion

Corrosion is the involuntary breakdown of metals by an electrochemical reaction and through the loss of ions from the metal surface in an acidic, an alkaline or a neutral environment. It is one of the most common reasons for implant failure [98]. **Table 3** summarises the types of corrosions that have been observed in metal implants [98–100].

Magnesium for example corrodes faster with an increase of impurities such as nickel, copper and iron [101]. The higher the purity of magnesium, the slower its corrosion rate. However, pure magnesium is not suitable for medical implants due to its mechanical characteristics. Instead, calcium is used for the grain refinement in magnesium alloys [102]. Orthopaedic implants fabricated from Mg-Ca alloys were observed to corrode over a 3-month period after bone formation [103]. Magnesium's mechanical properties can also be enhanced through Mg-Zn with calcium, manganese, yttrium or zirconium [104, 105]. Mg-Zn alloys withstand galvanic corrosion and biocorrosion *in vitro*; however, biocorrosion *in vivo* resulted in a 2 mm/year reduction of a Mg-Zn alloy used as rods in femur shafts [106].

3.2.2 Polymer degradation

Polymer degradation, or biodegradation, occurs through a process called hydrolysis. The polymer surface is attacked by organisms, which secrete enzymes breaking down ester bonds in macromolecules. The resulting smaller polymer molecules are further converted into carbon dioxide and water. The process of biodegradation varies for each polymer [27, 107, 108]; however, all polymers lose their mechanical integrity. To date, PGA, PLA and PLGA among others have been explored for biomedical implants [27]. Their degradation into non-toxic by-products made them favourable materials for temporary biomedical implants [109]. Poly(L-lactic) acid

Corrosion type	Explanation	Biomedical implants
Crevice corrosion	• Occurs in narrow regions • Metal ions create localised positive charge in the crevice	• Interfaces between screws/plates and bone
Pitting corrosion	• Occurs in implants with small surface pit • Metal ions react with chloride ions resulting in rough surfaces	• Orthopaedic and dental implants
Galvanic corrosion	• Occurs due to electrical gradient between Co-Cr alloys, Ni-Cr, Ag-Pd, Au-ternary Ti	• Oral/dental implants • Screws and nuts
Corrosion fatigue and fretting	• Occurs due to cyclic stress	• Bone cement • Femoral implants • Bone plates and screws at the bone-stem interface • Stem-cement interfaces of modular hip implant

Table 3.
Types of corrosions observed in metallic biomedical implants.

(PLLA) has been shown to induce inflammatory responses *in vivo* upon degradation due to its high crystallinity; hence, poly(D, L-lactic acid) (PDLA) was synthesised [110, 111].

PLGA degrades into acidic moieties, which in higher concentrations can affect the microenvironment of the implant's surrounding tissue. This can be especially important for drug delivery applications, where pH-sensitive drugs are used [11]. By increasing the amount of poly(glycolic acid) (PGA) compared to poly(lactic acid) (PLA) in PLGA, the degradation rate is reduced; hence, less acidic by-products are formed [11].

3.3 Biocompatibility

Biocompatibility indicates a desired response of the implant to its biological surrounding [34] and depends on biodegradability and corrosion. The ISO 10993 standard series is used to assess biocompatibility of medical grade materials and medical devices [112]. Test categories investigate the materials' cytotoxicity, sensitization, irritation, toxicity, implantation and biodegradation [71]. Materials that meet these criteria include noble metals and titanium, their alloys, cobalt-based alloys, but also alumina, zirconia, quartz, fused silica, bioglass, silicon, biocompatible polymers like epoxies, silicones, polyurethanes, polyimides, silicon-polyimides, polycyclic-olefins, silicon-carbons, and liquid crystal polymers [113].

3.4 Foreign body response

Foreign body response (FBR) is a non-specific immune reaction of the body to implanted materials. This inflammatory reaction can happen in response to surgical implantation of biodegradable or non-biodegradable materials present in medical devices or implants [114, 115]. FBR can modulate the safety and/or function of the implanted material. FBR is characterised by distinct phases, namely onset, progression and resolution [116] (**Figure 1**). The onset starts with the surgical implantation of the biomaterial, for example, subcutaneously, which causes local tissue damage [117]. Upon tissue damage, vessel permeation to cells and proteins increases and coagulation occurs where inflammatory mediators like vascular endothelial growth factor (VEGF) plays an important role along with neutrophils and macrophages to initiate the wound healing process. In parallel, angiogenic factors stimulate local vasculature.

FBR comprises of a biomaterial-dependent and biomaterial-independent reaction (**Figure 1**). If biodegradable materials are present, the FBR will persist until the material is fully degraded. With non-degradable or long-term implants, a fibrotic capsule creating a barrier between the material and the body will form.

Progression of FBR depends on the material's surface chemistry and wettability [118], where protein, antibody and macrophage adsorption can vary due to the material's intrinsic properties. Additionally, fibrinogen can be adsorbed by the implant altering its structure. During FBR's progression, leukocyte extraversion occurs from the blood vessels. These migrate towards the foreign body. Consequently, polymorphonuclear neutrophils (PMNs) are activated, which recruit cells including macrophages to the site. Macrophage activation leads to the recruitment of fibroblasts, monocytes and more PMNs [116], which ultimately increases production of extracellular matrix and hence implant encapsulation and fibrosis.

Phagocytosis occurs from the onset when antibodies are non-specifically adsorbed by the biomaterials, thus recruiting phagocytes. During progression,

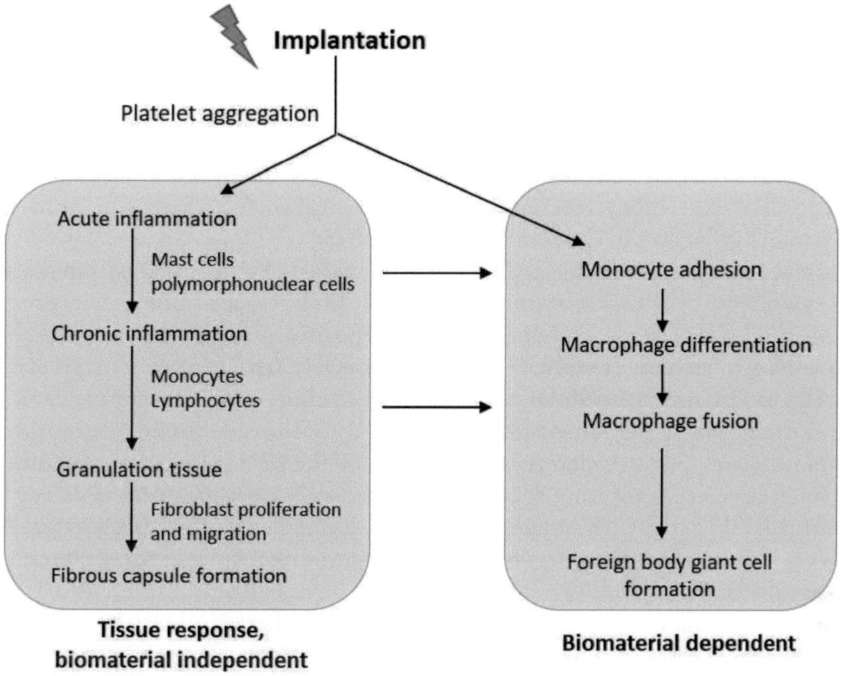

Figure 1.
Foreign body response to implant materials. Sequence of events and responses leading to the fibrous capsule formation and foreign body giant cell formation (adapted from [117]).

phagocytosis by macrophages is continuously promoted through the degradation of the material through biodegradation.

Material particles too large to be phagocyted cause the formation of larger multinucleated cells by fusion of macrophages. These so-called foreign body giant cells possess an irregular shape with more than 20 nuclei dispersed randomly. Giant cells will usually disappear once the foreign body is fully degraded. Surface roughness and surface/volume ratio of the implant can influence the adhesion of macrophages or prevalence of fibrosis [114].

As part of FBR, fibrosis is critical in tissue engineering, since capsule formation can prevent the diffusion of molecules (e.g., drugs) and continuous fibrosis formation can lead to capsule shrinkage thus affecting the implant structure [119]. It has been shown that inhibition of TGF-β can reduce capsule formation [120].

Finally, resolution of the foreign body response involves the degradation of the biomaterial or removal of the non-degradable material.

3.4.1 Immunomodulation for circumventing the foreign body response

Biomaterials' characteristics partly determine the body's immune response to the implant. Implant pore size and morphology are critical since they can allow immune cells and macromolecules to interact with the implant. In addition, degradation products derived from implants like scaffolds and medical devices, as well as their constantly changing surfaces, can trigger the immune response [121]. Recent implants can carry therapeutic cells. These cellular implants provoke an immune response due to encapsulated cells, posing further challenges besides biomaterial compatibility and design [122–124].

Polymers such as collagen, alginate, chitosan, polyethylene glycol, polyvinyl alcohol and polyurethane are used in several implantable products that may have an inherent biocompatibility. Understanding how these polymer's chemical and physical properties can be used to either avoid immune response or modulate it, while improving their functionality, is crucial for the advancement of these systems [121].

Strategies to circumvent the FBR include changing the biomaterial's surface properties like wettability, its chemical moieties, and surface charge, because they affect protein adhesion to the biomaterial [121, 125].

To create more hydrophilic surfaces, monolayers of hydrophilic polymers such as polyethylene glycol (PEG) and polyethylene oxide (PEO) are added, thus preventing protein adsorption altogether [126]. The deposition of chemical moieties like amino ($-NH_2$), carboxyl ($-COOH$), hydroxyl ($-OH$), and methyl ($-CH_3$) groups allows the modulation of cellular adhesion influencing inflammatory cell infiltration and macrophage response affecting the fibrotic capsule thickness around the implant [121]. Surface charge is important for the FBR immunomodulation. There have been contradicting reports on how exactly neutral, positive or negative charges reduce the inflammatory response connected to the FBR. Generally, negatively charged surfaces tend to inhibit the immune response through reduced cell adhesion [127].

Moreover, implant topography including texture, shape and size has shown to trigger an FBR [121]. Therefore, several manufacturing techniques like particles, assembled monolayers and photolithography are used to create variety of shapes, sizes and surface topographies [128, 129]. Surface roughness at the nanoscale can modulate protein adsorption [130], while variations in surface roughness at microscale affect cells directly [131]. For example, the inflammatory response of titanium used for dental or orthopaedic applications can be decreased by altering its surface nano-and microstructures via physical or chemical procedures [121].

Macrophage interaction with differently shaped biomaterials demonstrated preferred internalisation of nanorods via pinocytosis compared to nanospheres. Additionally, sharper cornered surfaces led to more acute immune responses than smoother surfaces [121, 132]. Moreover, spherical alginate capsules of 1.5 mm or greater were reported to be more biocompatible than their smaller, non-spherical comparators, demonstrating that larger, rounder, smoother capsules could diminish the FBR [133].

The use of decellularised ECM as scaffolds by removing immunogenic components to avoid an acute response but keeping the original structure has been studied. While decellularised ECMs contribute to a pro-regenerative environment [134], it has been discussed that the immune response modulation still depends on the original tissue from which the ECMs have been obtained. Therefore, this option still presents a potential solution with more research needed to advance its understanding, manufacturing and impact [134].

The incorporation of bioactive molecules such as adhesion molecules, drugs and growth factors to promote immunological interaction with the host attenuating its response has been investigated. Bioactive molecules bound to the biomaterial for controlled release aiding tissue regeneration [125] include proinflammatory molecules like prostaglandins [135] and anti-inflammatory molecules like cytokines [136]. Combining their delivery with glucocorticoids improved tissue regeneration and attenuation of inflammation [137]. In recent years, the encapsulation of immune cells that act as producers or inducers of specific biological responses to reduce inflammation and/or induce repair has been investigated as immunomodulation strategy [125]. Examples include the encapsulation of MSCs to decrease the fibrosis in FBR [138] or the encapsulation of macrophages to mediate pro-angiogenic activation [139].

Overall, understanding the fundamental biological systems associated with FBR and the structural, physical and chemical properties of biomaterials will lead to new designs and strategies allowing to circumvent or work together with the natural body's response towards implants.

4. Bioactive implants

Implants can be bioactive, inducing an alteration to the surrounding tissue, by their own biomaterials imparting this alteration to the surrounding tissue, by releasing a drug (or drugs) inducing bioactivity, or by containing cells that can produce bioactive molecules. In the following sub-sections, we discuss the implant bioactivity induced by drugs and cells implicating in drug delivery and in tissue regeneration.

4.1 Bioactive implantable and injectable drug delivery systems

Bioactive implants may incorporate active substances including small chemicals, peptides, proteins, hormones and even cells, which will have a therapeutic function in the human body. For drug delivery, these systems are commonly administered via parenteral route by injection or implantation. There are also implantable drug delivery systems that can be administered via ocular administration or via surgical procedures such as brain implants (e.g., Gliadel®). Implantable drug delivery systems are designed to slowly release the active substance(s) that they carry, thus avoiding repetitive injection. The active substance is delivered at a consistent predictable rate creating a drug release profile. This avoids peaks and troughs in the drug-blood level, which is common for non-long acting injectable products (e.g., intravenous solutions). Implantable drug delivery systems can be also injected subcutaneously, intramuscular or via other sites including intra-articular. They include implants and suspensions of micro- or nano-particles. Typically, these systems are preferred when the active substance has a poor absorption by other means of administration or a short half-life. The major advantages of such systems are improved pharmacokinetics, control of the drug release rate, and enhanced patient acceptability due to the reduction of side effects by maintaining the drug-blood level constant and by decreasing administration frequency [140, 141].

Sustained drug release is obtained via diffusion of the active substance through a biomaterial matrix, or released through biomaterial biodegradation, or a combination of both mechanisms. To date, commonly used biomaterials for drug delivery are either biodegradable like PCL and PLA or non-biodegradable like polydimethylsiloxane, polyethyl vinyl acetate, or titanium alloy [141]. Several approaches have been developed to produce implantable drug delivery systems [142] and to control the drug release. These include (i) using diffusion via membrane permeation, either porous or semi-porous membranes; (ii) controlling drug release by matrix diffusion using porous polymers; (iii) reservoir systems, where the drug is encapsulated in an inner reservoir; and (iv) actively releasing the drug from the implant via osmotic pressure, electric current, vapour pressure, hydrolysis or ultrasound activation.

Typically, simple rod-like solid implants, produced by hot melt extrusion processes using biodegradable polymers like PLA, PCL, PLGA and PEVA, often display a biphasic drug release kinetics showing a burst release due to the drug being deposited on the surface or near the surface of the implant, followed by a zero-order kinetics reflected by drug diffusion, matrix erosion, or a combination of both depending on the polymeric biomaterial used. **Table 4** summarises drug release systems that are currently commercially available or

System	Product	Drug	Manufacturer	Indication	Clinical status
Implants [143–148]	Zoladex® (PLGA solid rod, 1 × 10 mm)	Goserelin (up to 3 month release)	AstraZeneca	Prostate cancer	Approved by FDA
	Nexplanon® (radiopaque PEVA solid rod)	Etonogestrel (release up to 3 years)	Merck	Contraception	Approved by FDA
	ITCA 650 (Medici technology, former Duros®)	Exenatide (release up to 2 years)	Ipsen	Type 2 diabetes	Clinical Phase III/ NDA
	MK-8591 (PCL solid implant)	EFdA (long-term release)	Merck	HIV treatment and prevention	Pre-clinical/Phase I
Microparticles [149–151]	Risperdal Consta® (PLGA microspheres)	Risperidone	Janssen	Antipsychotic	Approved by FDA
	Decapeptyl SR® (PLGA microspheres)	Triptorelin	Debiopharm/Ferring/ Ipsen	Prostate cancer	Approved by FDA
	Sandostatin LAR® (PLGA microspheres)	Octreotide	Novartis	Acromegaly	Approved by FDA
	Bydureon® (PLGA microspheres)	Exenatide	Amylin/AstraZeneca	Type 2 diabetes	Approved by FDA
	Vivitrol® (PLGA microspheres)	Naltrexone	Alkermes	Opioid/alcohol dependence	Approved by FDA
In situ hydrogels [152, 153]	Eligard® (Atrigel® technology)	Leuprolide acetate	Sanofi-Aventis	Prostate cancer	Approved by FDA
	Posidin® (Sabre® technology)	Bupivacaine	Durect/Sandoz	Postoperative pain	Clinical Phase III/ NDA
	Relday® (Sabre® technology)	Risperidone	Durect/Zogenix	Schizophrenia/bipolar disorder	Phase I
	Sublocade® (Atrigel® technology)	Buprenorphine	Indivior	Severe opioid use disorder	Approved by FDA

Summarised are current systems that are commercially available or under development. Table was adapted from [140, 141, 148, 151, 153].

Table 4.
Drug delivery systems as implantable and injectable depots.

under development. There are numerous advantages to using implants in drug delivery such as the possibility of removal after treatment, the consistent and predictable drug release, and versatility in manufacture using various biomaterials. However, there are potential disadvantages of this dosage form, where often a specialised device (e.g., trocar) and technique are needed for implantation and removal requires minor surgical procedures. Additionally, there may be complications in locating the implant for removal since it can migrate from its original location. From a commercialisation point of view, this type of bioactive implant may require complex regulatory and commercial strategies for market approval [154].

Injectable drug delivery systems, such as particulate suspensions or hydrogels like *in situ* forming gel depots, are designed from biodegradable biomaterials, injected (e.g., subcutaneous, intramuscular), form a depot, erode when in contact with body fluids, and release the drug by diffusion and erosion [149]. Injectable depots are not designed to be retrieved. Examples of injectable depots are micro- or nano-scale particles, where the drug is encapsulated within the polymer matrix. The polymeric particles are commonly prepared from biodegradable materials (e.g., PLGA, PCL, or silica) since the intent is to deliver the depot system once by injection, let it erode and release the drug with time.

Choosing the polymer grade, type and combining polymer types can help tune the drug release as necessary [149, 154]. Key points in preparing these bioactive depots are the choice of the biomaterial (biodegradable/erodible), the physicochemical properties of drug to be encapsulated (i.e., hydrophobic or hydrophilic), the drug loading needed to deliver the therapeutic dose, and the inherent pharmacokinetics of the drug. This will inform the choice of manufacturing methods, often by emulsification. Common polymers used in these preparations are PLGA and PLA, where their long safety records deem these polymers as preferred, even though some minor inflammatory responses can still be reported [150].

Hydrogels, prepared from different types of biomaterials (e.g., hyaluronic acid, polyesters and chitosan) have been extensively investigated as carriers for sustained drug release [152, 155]. *In situ* forming hydrogels as injectable depots pose major advantages over other drug release systems since they allow for rapid, painless and easier administration through smaller needle sizes. These biodegradable *in situ* depots are of low viscosity prior injection and solidify into a gel or solid depot after injection, typically due to a specific trigger depending on the chemistry of the chosen biomaterial [153].

4.2 Bioactive cell-based implants as drug delivery systems

Before commercialising a cellular implant, it needs to be approved by FDA's Cellular, Tissue and Gene Therapies Advisory Committee. The Committee evaluates the safety and effectiveness of cellular implants for the reconstruction, repair or replacement of damaged tissues [156].

Cell-based drug delivery systems can be defined as technologies capable of treating diseases using living cells to deliver the therapeutic bioactive molecules in the body, as either transport system or as production units [157]. Some examples of commercially available or under development cell-based implants are shown in **Table 5**. These cell-based drug delivery systems are used as constant producers of bioactive molecules in the form of implant devices. Judging by the current developments in this technology, a major driving force behind this type of delivery is the improvement in treatment of insulin-dependent diabetes mellitus. The biggest challenge in cell-based drug delivery systems is avoiding immune response.

Company	Product	Application	Method of action	Manufacture
Neurotech	Encapsulated cell therapy (ECT)	Ophthalmology	Ciliary neurotrophic factor (CNTF) has neuroprotective effects on photoreceptors.	Encapsulated human cells producing CNTF into the back of the eye.
VIaCyte	Encaptra®	Stem cell delivery for treatment of diabetes mellitus	Human stem cells are isolated and differentiated into β islet cells contained into a pouch, which is implanted.	PTFE porous membrane device filled with cells.
Sernova	Cell Pouch™ with Sertolin™	Diabetes/haemophilia/thyroid disease	Therapeutic cells are inserted into a pouch made of medical-grade materials inserted subcutaneously; Sertolin® is a patented immune protection system.	Pouch made of medical-grade materials.
PharmaCyte	Cell-in-a-box®	Pancreatic cancer/breast cancer/diabetes	Uses cotton cellulose to encapsulate cells.	Single cell encapsulation in proprietary polymer, freeze-drying process to keep cells viable in the long term.
Beta-O2	βAir® bioartificial pancreas	Diabetes, adrenal insufficiency	Device using alginate—high guluronic acid and high mannuronic acid—to encapsulate cells and impregnate a PTFE porous membrane, respectively. Also comprises an oxygen-providing chamber, which needs refilling.	Single cell encapsulation in proprietary polymer, freeze-drying process to keep cells viable in the long term.
Sigilon	Afibromer™	Diabetes	Human stem cells differentiated to β islets encapsulated in modified alginate spheres, which suppress immune system response and FBR.	
Encapsulife	Encapsulation system for the immunoisolation of living cells	Diabetes	Cellulose-based polymer encapsulation of cells.	Pancreatic islets encapsulated are stimulated to produce insulin.
Organogenesis incorporated	GINTUIT	Mucogingival conditions	Keratinocytes and fibroblasts produce cytokines and growth factors that promote healing and regeneration of the tissue.	Allogeneic keratinocytes and fibroblast in bovine collagen.

Table 5.
Examples of commercially available cell-based implants for drug delivery.

4.3 Bioactive cellular implants as tissue replacements

When damages due to disease, injury or trauma lead to the degeneration of tissues, it is necessary to provide support for their repair, replacement or regeneration. Common approaches include tissue transplantation, both from the patient's own body (autograft) and from a donor (allograft). However, harvesting autografts is expensive and invasive and the patient may experience infections and hematomas. While for the allografts, there are risks of rejection along with the infections due to the surgery or the transplanted tissue [158]. With tissue engineering, biological implants are developed that restore, maintain and improve the tissue function [159]. Implants provide the environment for cell adhesion and proliferation to grow new tissues. They can also include active substances like growth factors and drugs as well as cells to aid tissue regeneration [11]. Cell-based scaffolds are either cultured *in vitro* with the aim of synthetizing tissues that can be implanted, or to be implanted directly in the damaged region [158]. **Table 6** summarises some of the recent studies about cell-based implants tested on *in vivo* models.

4.3.1 Primary cells versus stem cells

The advantage of using cell-based scaffolds is the possibility to customise the construct using cells derived from the patient (primary cells). In this way, there is no risk of rejection due to immunological incompatibility. Cells can be isolated from biopsies and then seeded on the scaffold (**Figure 2**). However, primary cells are differentiated, post-mitotic cells. This leads to a limited lifespan, where after a limited number of cell doubling, they will enter in senescence and stop dividing, but are still viable [166, 167]. Moreover, primary cell types are difficult to culture, because they have difficulties adhering and proliferating *in vitro* [168].

To overcome problems associated with primary cells, stem cells have been be used. Stem cells are present in most if not all tissues and, according to their origin, they can be classified into embryonic and adult stem cells. Stem cells are able to both duplicate (self-renew) and differentiate in one or more cell types [167].

Embryonic stem cells (ESCs) are isolated from inner cell mass of embryo at the blastocyst stage. They can differentiate in any cell type (pluripotency) and have a high rate of self-renewal. Unfortunately, they can cause an immune response, as they are derived from a different body, so immunosuppression is necessary to avoid rejection. Moreover, the injection of undifferentiated ESC can lead to the formation of teratoma [169].

Adult stem cells (ASCs) are multipotent cells that can differentiate in a limited number of cell types, which reside in a specific microenvironment, the stem cell niche. Their role is to replace damaged and dead cells in the tissue to maintain homeostasis [170].

ASCs can be isolated from bone marrow, blood, adipose tissue, liver and skin [169]. Compared to ESCs, ASCs proliferate more slowly and have limited expansion capacity *in vitro*. Like primary cells, they can enter in senescence [171]. With age, their regenerative potential, growth and divisions are affected [172]. The most commonly used type of ASCs is mesenchymal stem cells (MSCs). These cells can differentiate into musculoskeletal cells, marrow and other cells of connective tissue, and they can provide trophic support and modulate the immune response [173]. They can migrate to a damaged region and promote healing by secreting molecules involved in angiogenesis and cell proliferation and inhibit oxidative stress and apoptosis [174, 175].

Application	Cell type	Implant	Outcome	Reference
Tendon regeneration	Rat tendon stem/progenitor cells	Asymmetric chitosan-based sponges	• Tenogenic specific genes expression and protein production *in vitro* and *in vivo*. • Formation of aligned collagen fibres *in vivo*.	[160]
Neural tissue engineering	Schwann cells, human bone marrow mesenchymal stem cells (BMSCs)	Polyvinyl alcohol (PVA)/sulphate alginate nanofibers	• Metabolic active cells adhered to scaffold. • Mesenchymal stem cells differentiate in neuronal cells.	[161]
Wound healing and skin regeneration	Wharton's jelly mesenchymal stem cells (MSCs)	Poly(ε-caprolactone) (PCL)/gelatin nanofibers	• Nanofibrous biodegradable scaffolds. • Cells were metabolic active and proliferative after 21 days in culture. • MSCs on the scaffolds reduced the presence of denaturised proteins *in vitro*, possible anti-inflammatory response.	[162]
Mandible defects repair	Endothelial progenitor cells (EPCs), BMSCs	Biodegradable bioactive glass ceramic scaffold	• Expression of osteogenesis and angiogenesis markers *in vitro*. • After 9 months post-implantation *in vivo*, the defects were nearly completely recovered, and angiogenesis was promoted.	[163]
Acute kidney injury	Human placenta-derived mesenchymal stem cells (hP-MSCs)	Self-assembling peptide hydrogel	• hP-MSCs niche, cell survival and angiogenesis were promoted in *in vivo*. • Renal functions were ameliorated.	[164]
Spinal cord regeneration	Neural stem cells (NSCs)	Elastic poly(sebacoyl diglyceride) (PSeD) scaffolds coated with poly(sebacoyl diglyceride)-isoleucine-lysinevaline-alanine-valine-serine (PSeD-IKVAVS)	• Graft-host integration in spinal cord *in vivo*. • NSCs exhibited neuronal differentiation. • Inflammatory cells infiltrated the lesion site, functional recovery after 4 weeks. • Degradation products of PSeD-IKVAVS promoted NSCs differentiation, inhibited neuronal apoptosis and alleviated inflammation.	[165]

Table 6.
Examples of recent studies on cell-based implants.

Induced pluripotent stem cells (iPSCs) originate from fully differentiated somatic cells, which are dedifferentiated to form iPSCs by a process called reprogramming. The methodology was developed in 2006 [176] and involves the stimulation of genes that are active during the embryogenesis. Thanks to the cell derivation, the implantation of these cells does not lead to rejection. However, as with ESCs, iPSCs can form teratoma. Moreover, some of the genes that are activated are also associated with tumour development [177].

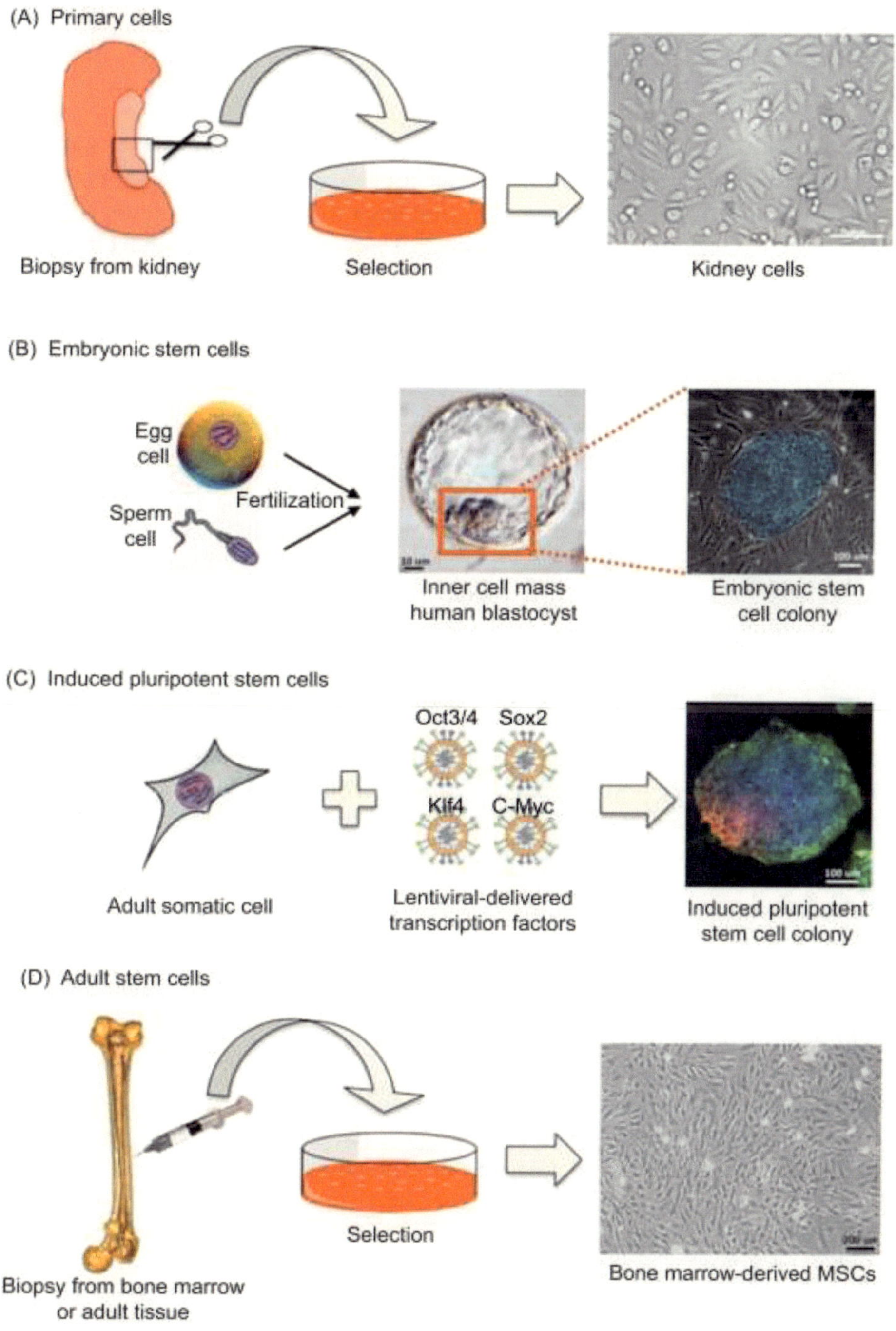

Figure 2.
Source of cells used for cell-based implants. Image adapted from [168].

5. Implant manufacture

To generate tissue replacements, it is essential to resemble the native extracellular matrix (ECM). Therefore, the matrix composition, shape and physical properties are crucial. Nanofibers, sponges or gels have been fabricated using numerous different techniques or combinations of techniques to mimic the native ECMs. Some of these techniques and their biomedical applications are presented in **Table 7**.

5.1 Solvent casting particulate leaching

Solvent casting particulate leaching is a technique developed in 1993 by Mikos et al., where a polymer is dissolved in an organic solvent and the polymer solution is mixed with an insoluble porogen. The solvent is evaporated by solvent casting or freeze-drying techniques. The evaporation leads to a porogen-polymer compound, which is washed to remove the porogen leaving a porous polymer matrix behind [187, 188]. This method is relatively easy to use and inexpensive [189]. Pore size, porosity and interconnectivity can be controlled selecting the right polymer, porogen and their concentration [190].

5.2 Phase separation

Phase separation employs temperature changes that separate the polymeric solution in two phases: the lean phase (low polymer concentration) and the rich phase (high polymer concentration). Briefly, the polymer is dissolved in a solvent, then, the temperature is rapidly decreased to have a liquid-liquid separation and two-phase solid is formed [191]. Finally, the liquid is removed by extraction, evaporation or sublimation [192].

5.3 Freeze-drying

Freeze-drying technique or lyophilisation [193] is based on a sublimation process that will produce a porous scaffold. A polymer is added to a mixture of water and organic solvent and moved into a mould. The mixture is quickly frozen and, by lowering the pressure to few millibars, the water and the organic solvent sublimate. The complete removal of the liquid phase takes place under vacuum [189, 194, 195]. To control porosity and pore size, polymer/water ratio, ionic concentration, viscosity and pH, together with freezing rate and temperature, can be changed [194, 195].

5.4 Electrospinning

Electrospinning is used to produce micro- and nanofibers. It is widely used as it can produce matrix that can resemble the native ECMs. Nanofiber scaffolds offer mechanical support and a nanoscale environment for the cells [196, 197]. A polymer solution is added to a syringe. Then, high voltage is applied, and the solution accelerates to a collector of opposite charge. The solution-air interface changes from rounded to conical, due to the repulsive electrostatic forces between the polymer molecules in solution and the attractive force between the polymer solution and the collector. The polymer solution is ejected from the syringe when the electrostatic forces are higher than the surface tension of the solution. Then, the solvent evaporates, and the solid polymer is deposited

Technique	Material	Application	Outcome	References
Solvent casting—particulate leaching	Poly(L-lactic acid) (PLLA) and matrilin-3 (MATN3)	Articular cartilage regeneration	• Nanofibrous porous scaffold. • Cell hypertrophy and endochondral ossification prevented *in vivo*. • Chondrogenesis is promoted *in vivo*.	[178]
Phase separation—particulate leaching	Poly(lactic acid) (PLA)	Bone tissue engineering	• Porous scaffold. • Osteosarcoma cells (MG63) were metabolic active and viable after 14 days in culture.	[179]
Freeze-drying	Poly(ε-caprolactone) (PCL) and zein	Drug delivery	• Porous and degradable scaffold. • Degradation rate increases with the concentration of zein.	[180]
Freeze-drying and self-assembly	Collagen	Tissue engineering	• Aligned collagen scaffolds. • Rat fibroblasts and neurons elongate along aligned fibres.	[181]
Freeze-drying	Silk fibroin-chitosan	Cartilage regeneration	• Porous scaffold. • MSCs were metabolic active, viable and differentiate after 21 days in culture.	[182]
Electrospinning	Poly(ε-caprolactone) (PCL)/poly(D,L-lactide-co-glycolide) (PLGA)/gelatin	Vascular tissue engineering	• Dual-oriented/bilayer hydrophilic nanofibers. • Smooth muscle cells and endothelial cells were viable after 7 days; orientation along the fibres.	[183]
Electrospinning	SiO_2CaO	Wound healing	• Cotton wool-like, fibrous and porous scaffold. • Human fibroblast seeded on top were metabolic active and proliferative after 7 days in culture, and produced vascular endothelial growth factor.	[184]
3D printing	Copper/tetrakis (4-carboxyphenyl) porphyrin/β-tricalcium phosphate (Cu-TCPP-TCP)	Bone tumour ablation and osteogenesis	• Metal-organic photothermal nanosheets. • Promoted osteosarcoma cell death *in vitro,* ablation of subcutaneous bone tumour tissue *in vivo*. • Adhesion of bone marrow MSCs HUVEC *in vitro*. • MSCs differentiated in osteocytes. • HUVEC expressed angiogenesis markers *in vitro*. • Enhanced bone regeneration *in vivo*.	[185]
E-jet 3D printing	Poly(lactic-co-glycolic acid) and drugs (5-fluorouracil and NVP-BEZ235)	Drug delivery in orthotopic breast cancer	• Long-term drug release near the tumour site. • Less risk for normal tissue. • No need for several administrations.	[186]

Table 7.
Techniques used for the fabrication of bioactive implants.

on the collector. By changing the voltage, collector, polymer concentration and solvent, it is possible to control the size of the fibres [196, 198].

5.5 Additive manufacturing techniques

Additive manufacturing (AM) techniques, or solid freeform fabrications (SFFs), are based on the use of computer-aided design (CAD) to fabricate scaffolds. The CAD controls the layer-by-layer deposition of material. The advantage of these methods is the full control of the topography of the construct [196, 198].

Three-dimensional (3D) printing is a commonly used AM technique that was developed at the Massachusetts Institute of Technology in 1990s [198, 199]. The CAD is converted in a stereo lithography (STL) file and exported to the 3D printer to control the movement and deposition of the material.

This technique allows the inclusion of cells within the scaffold, as high temperature or solvents are not required for its production [200]. In recent years, 3D printing has been used to produce scaffolds and anatomically customised implants based on MRI and CT scans. The AM can be classified in three different approaches [201], namely laser-based (stereolithography, selective laser sintering, electron beam melting and binder jetting) [202–204], nozzle-based (fused deposition modelling and melt electrospinning writing) [204–208] and indirect 3D printing [209–211].

5.6 Injection moulding

Injection moulding is one of the most commonly used techniques for large-scale production of thermoplastic items. The plastic is melted and injected into a mould of desired shape. When the material solidifies, the mould is removed, and the finished part is extracted [212]. Metal constructs can also be fabricated with this technique. Metal injection moulding uses fine metal powders mixed with a binder and is injected with a conventional thermoplastic moulding machine. The binder is then removed, and the product is formed. This method allows the production of constructs with a sophisticate shape and higher mechanical properties [213].

5.7 Self-assembly

Self-assembly is the spontaneous formation of molecular units in supramolecular structures, without external intervention. These molecules interact through hydrogen bonding, van der Waals and electrostatic forces. Due to their biocompatibility and biodegradability, peptides are commonly used for self-assembly. Specific structure can be created by modifying the amino-acidic composition of the peptides [189, 214]. These nanostructures can be used in drug delivery and tissue engineering [215].

5.8 Manufacturing considerations

The manufacturing of bioactive implants, whether these are for tissue engineering or for drug delivery purposes, includes several common aspects. These include the manufacturing methods that are employed, the biomaterial source, use of solvents, scalability, the need for aseptic facilities or if final product sterilisation is preferred, and if a specifically designed device is needed to administer the implant.

Most importantly, the regulatory strategy for filing needs to be in place soon in product development to define all the data that are needed for submission. It is important to define if the bioactive implant will be considered a drug product, a medical device, or a combination product (drug-device), and in which markets should it be launched, as different markets have different regulations and requisites for the different categories.

Comprehensive reviews and discussions on the regulatory aspects for filing medical devices, and combination products in the biomedical field were reviewed [216–218]. Ragelle et al. provide an excellent perspective for nanoparticle-based biomaterials, its manufacture and regulatory outlook for biomedical engineering [219].

To enable the use in animals and humans, the sterilisation process is important. If the manufacturing method is simplified enough, the use of aseptic technique for manufacturing, using filters and a particulate-free environment, will be possible although costly and complex for significantly large-scale manufacturing. For devices where metals are used, sterilisation by moist or dry heat may be possible.

However, for implants that involve polymers or heat-sensitive bioactive molecules, the preferred sterilisation method is gamma-irradiation. The drawback of using this technique is the potential risk to polymer and/or bioactive molecule degradation, changing the release rate and potentially compromising the efficacy of the implant [150]. Depending on the biomaterial and bioactive molecule involved, there may be ways to avoid degradation upon gamma-irradiation, such as using an antioxidant mixed with the drug. Apart from aseptic conditions, gamma-irradiation of the final product remains the best solution but exposes one of the disadvantages of developing bioactive implants as it is still a costly technique bringing its own risks [220].

6. Summary

In this chapter, we reviewed the current literature about bioactive biomedical implants applicable to regenerative therapies and used in drug delivery. To generate new biomedical implants, biomaterials are continuously developed, either through entirely new or by combining advantageous properties of well-known and safe biomaterials to improve the application and effectiveness of implants. Thus, materials that enhance the natural response of the body and simultaneously provide support for cell adhesion and proliferation are required. Another field that has developed in recent years is cell-induced bioactivity, where cells are used in implants for tissue regeneration and disease treatment. While there are several manufacturing techniques to create application-specific bioactive implants, new technologies, such as additive manufacturing, bring advantages and versatility to the field.

Author details

Andrea Domingues Goncalves[1], Wendy Balestri[2] and Yvonne Reinwald[2*]

1 Pharmaceutical Development—Oral and Inhaled, Product Development and Supply, GlaxoSmithKline, Ware, United Kingdom

2 Department of Engineering, Nottingham Trent University, Nottingham, United Kingdom

*Address all correspondence to: yvonne.reinwald@ntu.ac.uk

References

[1] Regulation of medical implants. House of Commons—Evidence—HC 163-i. 2019. Available from: http://www.publications.parliament.uk/pa/cm201213/cmselect/cmsctech/uc163-i/uc16301.htm

[2] Huang Y, Van Dessel J, Martens W, Lambrichts I, Zhong WJ, Ma GW, et al. Sensory innervation around immediately vs. delayed loaded implants: A pilot study. International Journal of Oral Science. 2015;**7**:49

[3] Arsiwala A, Desai P, Patravale V. Recent advances in micro/nanoscale biomedical implants. Journal of Controlled Release. 2014;**189**(2014):25-45

[4] Takmakov P, Ruda K, Phillips KS, Isayeva IS, Krauthamer V, Welle CG. Rapid evaluation of the durability of cortical neural implants using accelerated aging with reactive oxygen species. Journal of Neural Engineering. 2015;**12**:026003

[5] Guo R, Merkel AR, Sterling JA, Davidson JM, Guelcher SA. Substrate modulus of 3D-printed scaffolds regulates the regenerative response in subcutaneous implants through the macrophage phenotype and Wnt signaling. Biomaterials. 2015;**73**:85-95

[6] Li J, Stachowski M, Zhang Z. Application of responsive polymers in implantable medical devices and biosensors. In: Switchable and Responsive Surfaces and Materials for Biomedical Applications. Cambridge, UK: Elsevier; 2015. pp. 259-298

[7] Bagga C, Erbe EM, Murphy JP, Freid JM, Pomrink GJ. Bioactive Spinal Implants and Method of Manufacture Thereof. U.S. Patent 8,715,353; 2014

[8] Klein MO, Schiegnitz E, Al-Nawas B. Systematic review on success of narrow-diameter dental implants. The International Journal of Oral & Maxillofacial Implants. 2014;**29**:43-54

[9] Yahyavi-Firouz-Abadi N, Menias CO, Bhalla S, Siegel C, Gayer G, Katz DS. Imaging of cosmetic plastic procedures and implants in the body and their potential complications. American Journal of Roentgenology. 2015;**204**:707-715

[10] Silva VV, Domingues RZ, Lameiras FS. Microstructural and mechanical study of zirconia-hydroxyapatite (ZH) composite ceramics for biomedical applications. Composites Science and Technology. 2001;**61**:301-310

[11] Stratton S, Shelke NB, Hoshino K, Rudraiah S, Kumbar SG. Bioactive polymeric scaffolds for tissue engineering. Bioactive Materials. 2016;**1**(2):93-108

[12] Dhandayuthapani B, Sakthikumar D. Biomedical Applications of Polymeric Materials and Composites. 1st ed. Weinheim, Germany: Wiley; 2017. pp. 1-20

[13] Jones AJ, Denning NT. Polymeric Biomaterials: Bio- and Ecocompatible Polymers, A Perspective for Australia. Department of Industry, Technology and Commerce; 1988. ISBN: 0642134618, 9780642134615

[14] ASM International. Overview of biomaterials and their use in medical devices. Handbook of Materials for Medical Devices. Cleveland, OH, USA: ASM International, Inc; 2003

[15] Zdrahala RJ, Zdrahala IJ. Biomedical applications of polyurethanes: A review of past promises, present realities, and a vibrant future. Journal of Biomaterials Applications. 1999;**14**(1):67-90

[16] Daebritz SH, Fausten B, Hermanns B, Schroeder J, Groetzner J, Autschbach R, et al. Introduction of a flexible polymeric heart valve prosthesis with special design for the aortic position. Circulation. 2003;**108**(10-Suppl. 1):II-135-II-139

[17] Zhu Y, Gao C, He T, Shen J. Endothelium regeneration on luminal surface of polyurethane vascular scaffold modified with diamine and covalently grafted with gelatin. Biomaterials. 2004;**25**(3):423-430

[18] Yuan Y, Ai F, Zang X, Zhuang W, Shen J, Lin S. Polyurethane vascular catheter surface grafted with zwitterionic sulfobetaine monomer activated by ozone. Colloids and Surfaces B. 2004;**35**(1):1-5

[19] Lin W-C, Tseng C-H, Yang M-C. In-vitro hemocompatibility evaluation of a thermoplastic polyurethane membrane with surfaceimmobilized water-soluble chitosan and heparin. Macromolecular Bioscience. 2005;**5**:1013-1021

[20] Topol EJ, Serruys PW. Frontiers in interventional cardiology. Circulation. 1802-1820;**1998**:98

[21] Whelan DM, van der Giessen WJ, Krabbendam SC, van Vliet EA, Verdouw PD, Serruys PW, et al. Biocompatibility of phosphorylcholine coated stents in normal porcine coronary arteries. Heart. 2000;**83**:338-345

[22] Horner PJ, Gage FH. Regenerating the damaged central nervous system. Nature. 2000;**407**:963-970

[23] Scheib J, Hoke A. Advances in peripheral nerve regeneration. Nature Reviews. Neurology. 2013;**9**:668-676

[24] Cao J, Xiao Z, Jin W, Chen B, Meng D, Ding W, et al. Induction of rat facial nerve regeneration by functional collagen scaffolds. Biomaterials. 2013;**34**:1302-1310

[25] White JD, Wang S, Weiss AS, Kaplan DL. Silke-tropoelastin protein films for nerve guidance. Acta Biomaterialia. 2015;**14**:1-10

[26] Xie J, MacEwan MR, Liu W, Jesuraj N, Li X, Hunter D, et al. Nerve guidance conduits based on double-layered scaffolds of electrospun nanofibers for repairing the peripheral nervous system. ACS Applied Materials & Interfaces. 2014;**6**:9472-9480

[27] Prakasam M, Locs J, Salma-Ancane K, Dagnija Loca D, Largeteau A, Berzina-Cimdina L. Biodegradable materials and metallic implants—A review. Journal of Functional Biomaterials. 2017;**8**:44

[28] Zimmerli W. Clinical presentation and treatment of orthopaedic implant-associated infection. Journal of Internal Medicine. 2014;**276**:111-119

[29] Bellini H, Moyano J, Gil J, Puigdollers A. Comparison of the superelasticity of different nickel–titanium orthodontic archwires and the loss of their properties by heat treatment. Journal of Materials Science. Materials in Medicine. 2016;**27**:158

[30] Hutmacher DW, Garcia AJ. Scaffold-based bone engineering by using genetically modified cells. Gene. 2005;**347**(1):1-10

[31] Liu YD, Hu J, Zhuang XL, et al. Synthesis and characterization of novel biodegradable and electroactive hydrogel based on aniline oligomer and gelatin. Macromolecular Bioscience. 2011;**12**:241-250

[32] Guo BL, Glavas L, Albertsson AC. Biodegradable and electrically

conducting polymers for biomedical applications. Progress in Polymer Science. 2013;**38**:1263-1286

[33] Guo BL, Finne-Wistrand A, Albertsson AC. Versatile functionalization of polyester hydrogels with electroactive aniline oligomers. Journal of Polymer Science Part A: Polymer Chemistry. 2011;**49**:2097-2105

[34] Saini M, Singh Y, Arora P, Arora V, Jain K. Implant biomaterials: A comprehensive review. World Journal of Clinical Cases. 2015;**3**(1): 52-57

[35] Sykaras N, Iacopino AM, Marker VA, Triplett RG, Woody RD. Implant materials, designs, and surface topographies: Their effect on osseointegration. A literature review. The International Journal of Oral & Maxillofacial Implants. 2000;**15**: 675-690

[36] LeGeros RZ, Lin S, Rohanizadeh R, Mijares D, LeGeros JP. Biphasic calcium phosphate bioceramics: Preparation, properties and applications. Journal of Materials Science. Materials in Medicine. 2003;**14**:201-209

[37] DeGroot K. Clinical applications of calcium phosphate biomaterials: A review. Ceramics International. 1993;**19**:363-366

[38] Wennerberg A, Albrektsson T. On implant surfaces: A review of current knowledge and opinions. The International Journal of Oral & Maxillofacial Implants. 2010;**25**:63-74

[39] Hoffmann O, Angelov N, Gallez F, Jung RE, Weber FE. The zirconia implant-bone interface: A preliminary histologic evaluation in rabbits. The International Journal of Oral & Maxillofacial Implants. 2008;**23**:691-695

[40] Özkurt Z, Kazazoğlu E. Zirconia dental implants: A literature review. The Journal of Oral Implantology. 2011;**37**:367-376

[41] Chiapasco M, Casentini P, Zaniboni M, Corsi E, Anello T. Titanium-zirconium alloy narrow-diameter implants (Straumann Roxolid(®)) for the rehabilitation of horizontally deficient edentulous ridges: Prospective study on 18 consecutive patients. Clinical Oral Implants Research. 2012;**23**:1136-1141

[42] Teramoto H, Kawai A, Sugihara S, Yoshida A, Inoue H. Resorption of apatite-wollastonite containing glass-ceramic and beta-tricalcium phosphate in vivo. Acta Medica Okayama. 2005;**59**:201-207

[43] Boanini E, Gazzano M, Bigi A. Ionic substitutions in calcium phosphates synthesized at low temperature. Acta Biomaterialia. 2010;**6**:1882-1894

[44] Thian ES, Konishi T, Kawanobe Y, Lim PN, Choong C, Ho B, et al. Zinc-substituted hydroxyapatite: A biomaterial with enhanced bioactivity and antibacterial properties. Journal of Materials Science. Materials in Medicine. 2013;**24**:437-445

[45] Mayer I, Jacobsohn O, Niazov T, Werckmann J, Iliescu M, Richard-Plouet M, et al. Manganese in precipitated hydroxyapatites. European Journal of Inorganic Chemistry. 2003:1445-1451

[46] Tamimi F, Le Nihouannen D, Eimar H, Sheikh Z, Komarova S, Barralet J. The effect of autoclaving on the physical and biological properties of dicalcium phosphate dihydrate bioceramics: Brushite vs. monetite. Acta Biomaterialia. 2012;**8**:3161-3169

[47] Hodosh M, Povar M, Shklar G. The dental polymer implant concept. The Journal of Prosthetic Dentistry. 1969;**22**:371-380

[48] Wang Y, Blasioli DJ, Kim H-J, Kim HS, Kaplan DL. Cartilage tissue engineering with silk scaffolds and human articular chondrocytes. Biomaterials. 2006;**27**:4434-4442

[49] Vepari C, Kaplan DL. Silk as a biomaterial. Progress in Polymer Science. 2007;**32**:991-1007

[50] Yang Y, Ding F, Wu J, Hu W, Liu W, Liu J, et al. Development and evaluation of silk fibroin-based nerve grafts used for peripheral nerve regeneration. Biomaterials. 2007;**28**:5526-5535

[51] Hakimi O, Knight DP, Vollrath F, Vadgama P. Spider and mulberry silkworm silks as compatible biomaterials. Composites. Part B, Engineering. 2007;**38**:324-337

[52] Etienne O, Schneider A, Kluge JA, Bellemin-Laponnaz C, Polidori C, Leisk GG, et al. Soft tissue augmentation using silk gels: An in vitro and in vivo study. Journal of Periodontology. 2009;**80**:1852-1858

[53] Kardestuncer T, McCarthy M, Karageorgiou V, Kaplan DL, Gronowicz G. RGD-tethered silk substrate stimulates the differentiation of human tendon cells. Clinical Orthopaedics and Related Research. 2006;**448**:234-239

[54] Cai Z-X, Mo X-M, Zhang K-H, Fan L-P, Yin A-L, He C-L, et al. Fabrication of chitosan/silk fibroin composite nanofibers for wound-dressing applications. International Journal of Molecular Sciences. 2010;**11**:3529-3539

[55] Okabayashi R, Nakamura M, Okabayashi T, Tanaka Y, Nagai A, Yamashita K. Efficacy of polarized hydroxyapatite and silk fibroin composite dressing gel on epidermal recovery from full-thickness skin wounds. Journal of Biomedical Materials Research Part B: Applied Biomaterials. 2009;**90B**:641-646

[56] Necas J, Bartosikova L, Brauner P, Kolar J. Hyaluronic acid (hyaluronan): A review. Veterinární Medicína. 2008;**53**:397-411

[57] Laurencin CT, Jiang T, Kumbar SG, Nair LS. Biologically active chitosan systems for tissue engineering and regenerative medicine. Current Topics in Medicinal Chemistry. 2008;**8**:354-364

[58] He S, Yaszemski MJ, Yasko AW, Engel PS, Mikos AG. Injectable biodegradable polymer composites based on poly (propylene fumarate) crosslinked with poly (ethylene glycol)-dimethacrylate. Biomaterials. 2000;**21**:2389-2394

[59] Shelke NB, Anderson M, Idrees S, Nip MJ, Donde S, Yu X, et al. Handbook of Polyester Drug Delivery Systems. Singapore: Pan Stanford; 2016. pp. 595-649

[60] Narayanan G, Gupta BS, Tonelli AE. Enhanced mechanical properties of poly(ε-caprolactone) nanofibers produced by the addition of nonstoichiometric inclusion complexes of poly(ε-caprolactone) and a-cyclodextrin. Polymer. 2015;**76**:321-330

[61] Karst D, Yang Y. Molecular modeling study of the resistance of PLA to hydrolysis based on the blending of PLLA and PDLA. Polymer. 2006;**47**:4845-4850

[62] Gentile P, Chiono V, Carmagnola I, Hatton PV. An overview of poly (lactic co-glycolic) acid (PLGA)-based biomaterials for bone tissue engineering. International Journal of Molecular Sciences. 2014;**15**:3640-3659

[63] Woodruff MA, Hutmacher DW. The return of a forgotten polymer

polycaprolactone in the 21st century. Progress in Polymer Science. 2010;**35**:1217-1256

[64] Nada AA, James R, Shelke NB, Harmon MD, Awad HM, Nagarale RK, et al. A smart methodology to fabricate electrospun chitosan nanofiber matrices for regenerative engineering applications. Polymers for Advanced Technologies. 2014;**25**:507-515

[65] Chang KY, Hung LH, Chu I, Ko CS, Lee YD. The application of type II collagen and chondroitin sulfate grafted PCL porous scaffold in cartilage tissue engineering. Journal of Biomedial Materials Research Part A. 2010;**92**:712-723

[66] Tan L, Yu X, Wan P, Yang K. Biodegradable materials for bone repairs: A review. Journal of Materials Science and Technology. 2013;**29**:503-513

[67] Pezzin AP, Ekenstein V, Alberda GO, Zavaglia CA, Ten Brinke G, Duek EA. Poly (para-dioxanone) and poly (L-lactic acid) blends: Thermal, mechanical, and morphological properties. Journal of Applied Polymer Science. 2003;**88**:2744-2755

[68] Amanatullah DF, Landa J, Strauss EJ, Garino JP, Kim SH, Di Cesare PE. Comparison of surgical outcomes and implant wear between ceramic-ceramic and ceramic-polyethylene articulations in total hip arthroplasty. Journal of Arthroplasty. 2011;**26**(6):72-77

[69] Green JM, Hallab NJ, Liao Y-S, Narayan V, Schwarz EM, Xie C. Anti-oxidation treatment of ultra high molecular weight polyethylene components to decrease periprosthetic osteolysis: Evaluation of osteolytic and osteogenic properties of wear debris particles in a murine calvaria model. Current Rheumatology Reports. 2013;**15**(5):1-5

[70] Zhou J, Huang X, Zheng D, Li H, Herrler T, Li Q. Oriental nose elongation using an L-shaped polyethylene sheet implant for combined septal spreading and extension. Aesthetic Plastic Surgery. 2014;**38**(2):295-302

[71] Teo AJT, Mishra A, Park I, Kim YJ, Park WT, Yoon YJ. Polymeric biomaterials for medical implants and devices. ACS Biomaterials Science & Engineering. 2016;**2**:454-472

[72] Pérez-Merino P, Dorronsoro C, Llorente L, Durán S, Jiménez-Alfaro I, Marcos S. In vivo chromatic aberration in eyes implanted with intraocular lenses. Investigative Ophthalmology & Visual Science. 2013;**54**(4):2654-2661

[73] Terrada C, Julian K, Cassoux N, Prieur A-M, Debre M, Quartier P, et al. Cataract surgery with primary intraocular lens implantation in children with uveitis: Long-term outcomes. Journal of Cataract & Refractive Surgery. 2011;**37**(11):1977-1983

[74] Kim B-J, Hong K-S, Park K-J, Park D-H, Chung Y-G, Kang S-H. Customized cranioplasty implants using three-dimensional printers and polymethyl-methacrylate casting. Journal of Korean Neurosurgical Association. 2012;**52**(6):541-546

[75] Rivkin A. A prospective study of non-surgical primary rhinoplasty using a polymethylmethacrylate injectable implant. Dermatologic Surgery. 2014;**40**(3):305-313

[76] Shklar G, Hodosh M, Povar M. Tissue reactions to polymer-coated vitallium pin implants. Journal of Prosthetic Dentistry. 1970;**24**:636-645

[77] Qin Y, Howlader MM, Deen MJ, Haddara YM, Selvaganapathy PR. Polymer integration for packaging of implantable sensors. Sensors and Actuators, B: Chemical. 2014;**202**:758

[78] Lachhman S, Zorman C, Ko W. Multi-layered polydimethylsiloxane as a non-hermetic packaging material for medical MEMS. In: 2012 Annual International Conference of the IEEE Engineering in Medicine and Biology Society (EMBC). Piscataway, NJ: IEEE; 2012. pp. 1655-1658

[79] Rahimi A, Mashak A. Review on rubbers in medicine: Natural, silicone and polyurethane rubbers. Plastics Rubber and Composites. 2013;**42**(6):223-230

[80] Kappel RM, Klunder AJ, Pruijn GJ. Silicon chemistry and silicone breast implants. European Journal of Plastic Surgery. 2014;**37**(3):123-128

[81] Kubyshkina G, Zupančič B, Štukelj M, GroŠelj D, Marion L, Emri I. Sterilization effect on structure, thermal and time-dependent properties of polyamides. In: Mechanics of Time-Dependent Materials and Processes in Conventional and Multifunctional Materials. Vol. 3. New York: Springer; 2011. pp. 11-19

[82] Cruz F. Fabrication of HA/PLLA composite scaffolds for bone tissue engineering using additive manufacturing technologies. In: Elnashar M, editor. Biopolymers. Rijeka, Croatia: INTECH Open Access; 2010. pp. 227-242. (Chapter 11)

[83] Li X, Liu X, Huang J, Fan Y, Cui, F.-z. Biomedical investigation of CNT based coatings. Surface and Coating Technology. 2011;**206**(4):759-766

[84] Li N, Zheng Y. Novel magnesium alloys developed for biomedical application: A review. Journal of Materials Science and Technology. 2013;**29**:489-502

[85] Witte F, Fischer J, Nellesen J, Crostack HA, Kaese V, Pisch A, et al. In vitro and in vivo corrosion measurements of magnesium alloys. Biomaterials. 2006;**27**:1013-1018

[86] Tang A, Pan F, Yang M, Cheng R. Mechanical properties and microstructure of magnesium-aluminum based alloys containing strontium. Materials Transactions. 2008;**49**:1203-1211

[87] Tekumalla S, Seetharaman S, Almajid A, Gupta M. Mechanical properties of magnesium-rare earth alloy systems: A review. Metals. 2015;**5**:1-39

[88] Taïr K, Kharoubi O, Taïr OA, Hellal N, Benyettou I, Aoues A. Aluminium-induced acute neurotoxicity in rats: Treatment with aqueous extract of Arthrophytum (*Hammada scoparia*). Journal of Acute Disease. 2016;**5**:470-482

[89] Gu X-N, Zheng Y-F. A review on magnesium alloys as biodegradable materials. Frontiers of Materials Science in China. 2010;**4**:111-115

[90] Zhang E, Yang L, Xu J, Chen H. Microstructure, mechanical properties and bio-corrosion properties of Mg–Si(–Ca, Zn) alloy for biomedical application. Acta Biomaterialia. 2010;**6**:1756-1762

[91] Kulkarni M, Mazare A, Gongadze E, Perutkova Š, Kralj-Igli V, Milošev I, et al. Titanium nanostructures for biomedical applications. Nanotechnology. 2015;**26**:062002

[92] Kopova I, Stráský J, Harcuba P, Landa M, Janeček M, Bačákova L. Newly developed Ti–Nb–Zr–Ta–Si–Fe biomedical beta titanium alloys with increased strength and enhanced biocompatibility. Materials Science and Engineering: C. 2016;**60**: 230-238

[93] Wang S, Liu Y, Zhang C, Liao Z, Liu W. The improvement of wettability,

biotribological behavior and corrosion resistance of titanium alloy pre-treated by thermal oxidation. Tribology International. 2014;**79**:174-182

[94] Li Y, Yang C, Zhao H, Qu S, Li X, Li Y. New developments of Ti-based alloys for biomedical applications. Materials. 2014;7:1709-1800

[95] Gepreel MA, Niinomi M. Biocompatibility of Ti-alloys for long-term implantation. Journal of the Mechanical Behavior of Biomedical Materials. 2013;**20**:407-415

[96] Arvidson K, Cottler-Fox M, Hammarlund E, Friberg U. Cytotoxic effects of cobalt-chromium alloys on fibroblasts derived from human gingiva. Scandinavian Journal of Dental Research. 1987;**95**:356-363

[97] Phillips RW. Skinner's Science of Dental Materials. 8th ed. Philadelphia: WB Saunders; 1982

[98] Manivasagam G, Dhinasekaran D, Rajamanickam A. Biomedical implants: Corrosion and its prevention—A review. Recent Patents on Corrosion Science. 2010;**2**:40-54

[99] Chaturvedi TP. An overview of the corrosion aspect of dental implants (titanium and its alloys). Indian Journal of Dental Research. 2009;**20**:91-98

[100] Adya N, Alam M, Ravindranath T, Mubeen A, Saluja B. Corrosion in titanium dental implants: Literature review. Journal of Indian Prosthodontic Society. 2005;**5**:126-131

[101] Song GL, Atrens A. Corrosion mechanisms of magnesium alloys. Advanced Engineering Materials. 1999;**1**:11-33

[102] Lee YC, Dahle AK, StJohn DH. Grain refinement of magnesium. In: Essential Readings in Magnesium Technology. Berlin, Germany: Springer; 2016. pp. 247-254

[103] Lee JW, Han HS, Han KJ, Park J, Jeon H, Ok MR, et al. Long-term clinical study and multiscale analysis of in vivo biodegradation mechanism of Mg alloy. Proceedings of the National Academy of Sciences of the United States of America. 2016;**113**:716-721

[104] Zhang S, Zhang X, Zhao C, Li J, Song Y, Xie C, et al. Research on an Mg–Zn alloy as a degradable biomaterial. Acta Biomaterialia. 2010;**6**:626-640

[105] Wang J, Zhang J, Zong X, Xu C, You Z, Nie K. Effects of Ca on the formation of LPSO phase and mechanical properties of Mg-Zn-Y-Mn alloy. Materials Science and Engineering A. 2015;**648**:37-40

[106] He Y, Tao H, Zhang Y, Jiang Y, Zhang S, Zhao C, et al. Biocompatibility of bio-Mg-Zn alloy within bone with heart, liver, kidney and spleen. Chinese Science Bulletin. 2009;**54**:484-491

[107] David C, De Kesel C, Lefebvre F, Weiland M. The biodegradation of polymers: Recent results. Macromolecular Materials and Engineering. 1994;**216**:21-35

[108] Premraj R, Doble M. Biodegradation of polymers. Indian Journal of Biotechnology. 2005;**4**:186-193

[109] Hule RA, Pochan DJ. Polymer nanocomposites for biomedical applications. MRS Bulletin. 2007;**32**: 354-358

[110] Lasprilla AJ, Martinez GA, Lunelli BH, Jardini AL, Maciel Filho R. Polylactic acid synthesis for application in biomedical devices: A review. Biotechnology Advances. 2012;**30**:321-328

[111] Fukushima K, Kimura Y. An efficient solid-state polycondensation method for synthesizing

stereo-complexed poly (lactic acid) s with high molecular weight. Journal of Polymer Science Part A: Polymer Chemistry. 2008;**46**:3714-3722

[112] Sastri VR. Plastics in Medical Devices: Properties, Requirements, and Applications. Cambridge, UK: William Andrew; 2013

[113] Joung Y-H. Development of implantable medical devices: From an engineering perspective. International Neurourology Journal. 2013;**17**(3):98-106

[114] Anderson J. Inflammatory response to implants. ASAIO Transactions. 1988;**34**(2):101-107

[115] Kenneth Ward W. A review of the foreign-body response to subcutaneously-implanted devices: The role of macrophages and cytokines in biofouling and fibrosis. Journal of Diabetes Science and Technology. 2008;**2**(5):768-777

[116] Luttikhuizen D, Harmsen M, Luyn M. Cellular and molecular dynamics in the foreign body reaction. Tissue Engineering. 2006;**12**(7):1955-1970

[117] Anderson J, Rodriguez A, Chang D. Foreign body reaction to biomaterials. Seminars in Immunology. 2008;**20**(2):86-100

[118] Wilson C, Clegg R, Leavesley D, Pearcy M. Mediation of biomaterial-cell interactions by adsorbed proteins: A review. Tissue Engineering. 2005;**11**(1-2):1-18

[119] Kuhn A, Singh S, Smit P, Ko F, Falcone R, Lyle W, et al. Periprosthetic breast capsules contain the fibrogenic cytokines TGF-beta1 and TGF-beta2, suggesting possible new treatment approaches. Annals of Plastic Surgery. 2000;**44**(4):387-391

[120] Mazaheri M, Schultz G, Blalock T, Caffee H, Chin G, Lineaweaver W. Role of connective tissue growth factor in breast implant elastomer capsular formation. Annals of Plastic Surgery. 2003;**50**(3):263-268

[121] Mariani E, Lisignoli G, Borzì R, Pulsatelli L. Biomaterials: Foreign bodies or tuners for the immune response? International Journal of Molecular Sciences. 2019;**20**(3):636-678

[122] Orive G, De Castro M, Kong H, Hernández R, Ponce S, Mooney D, et al. Bioactive cell-hydrogel microcapsules for cell-based drug delivery. Journal of Controlled Release. 2009;**135**(3):203-210

[123] Orive G, Santos E, Poncelet D, Hernández R, Pedraz J, Wahlberg L, et al. Cell encapsulation: Technical and clinical advances. Trends in Pharmacological Sciences. 2015;**36**(8):537-546

[124] Major M, Wong V, Nelson E, Longaker M, Gurtner G. The foreign body response: At the Interface of surgery and bioengineering. Plastic and Reconstructive Surgery. 2015;**135**(5):1489-1498

[125] Vishwakarma A, Bhise N, Evangelista M, Rouwkema J, Dokmeci M, Ghaemmaghami A, et al. Engineering immunomodulatory biomaterials to tune the inflammatory response. Trends in Biotechnology. 2016;**34**(6):470-482

[126] Drury J, Mooney D. Hydrogels for tissue engineering: Scaffold design variables and applications. Biomaterials. 2003;**24**(24):4337-4351

[127] Kakizawa Y, Lee J, Bell B, Fahmy T. Precise manipulation of biophysical particle parameters enables control of proinflammatory cytokine production in presence of TLR 3

and 4 ligands. Acta Biomaterialia. 2017;**15**(57):136-145

[128] Bota P, Collie A, Puolakkainen P, Vernon R, Sage E, Ratner B, et al. Biomaterial topography alters healing in vivo and monocyte/macrophage activation in vitro. Journal of Biomedical Materials Research. 2010;**95**(2):649-657

[129] Mohiuddin M, Pan H, Hung Y, Huang G. Control of growth and inflammatory response of macrophages and foam cells with nanotopography. Nanoscale Research Letters. 2012;**7**:394

[130] Scopelliti P, Borgonovo A, Indrieri M, Giorgetti L, Bongiorno G, Carbone R, et al. The effect of surface nanometre-scale morphology on protein adsorption. PLoS One. 2010;**5**(7):e11862

[131] Mrksich M, Whitesides G. Using self-assembled monolayers to understand the interactions of man-made surfaces with proteins and cells. Annual Review of Biophysics and Biomolecular Structures. 1996;**25**:55-78

[132] Bartneck M, Keul H, Singh S, Czaja K, Bornemann J, Bockstaller M, et al. Rapid uptake of gold nanorods by primary human blood phagocytes and immunomodulatory effects of surface chemistry. ACS Nano. 2010;**4**(6):3073-3086

[133] Veiseh O, Doloff J, Ma M, Vegas A, Tam H, Bader A, et al. Size- and shape-dependent foreign body immune response to materials implanted in rodents and non-human primates. Nature Materials. 2015;**14**:643-651

[134] Badylak S, Dziki J, Sicari B, Ambrosio F, Boninger M. Mechanisms by which acellular biologic scaffolds promote functional skeletal muscle restoration. Biomaterials. 2016;**103**:128-136

[135] Toyoda H, Terai H, Sasaoka R, Oda K, Takaoka K. Augmentation of bone morphogenetic protein-induced bone mass by local delivery of a prostaglandin E EP4 receptor agonist. Bone. 2005;**37**:555-562

[136] Wynn T, Vannella K. Macrophages in tissue repair, regeneration, and fibrosis. Immunity. 2016;**44**(3):450-462

[137] Tsianakas A, Varga G, Barczyk K, Bode G, Nippe N, Kran N, et al. Induction of an anti-inflammatory human monocyte subtype is a unique property of glucocorticoids, but can be modified by IL-6 and IL-10. Immunobiology. 2012;**217**(3):329-335

[138] Swartzlander M, Blakney A, Amer L, Hankenson K, Kyriakides T, Bryant S. Immunomodulation by mesenchymal stem cells combats the foreign body response to cell-laden synthetic hydrogels. Biomaterials. 2015;**41**:79-88

[139] Dohle E, Bischoff I, Bose T, Marsano A, Banfi A, Unger R, et al. Macrophage-mediated angiogenic activation of outgrowth endothelial cells in co-culture with primary osteoblasts. European Cells and Materials. 2014;**27**:149-164

[140] Tiwari G, Tiwari R, Bannerjee S, Bhati L, Pandey S, Pandey P, et al. Drug delivery systems: An updated review. International Journal of Pharmaceutical Investigation. 2012;**2**(1):2

[141] Koduri R, Mahalakshmi K, Maheswara Rao U. Implantable drug delivery systems: A review on parenteral implants. International Journal of Innovative Pharmaceutical Sciences and Research. 2015;**3**(9): 1406-1418

[142] Agrawal M, Limbachiya M, Sapariya A, Patel G. A review on

parenteral controlled drug delivery system. IJPSR. 2012;**3**(10):3657-3669

[143] Citrin D, Resnick M, Guinan P, Al-Bussam N, Scott M, Gau T, et al. A comparison of Zoladex@ and DES in the treatment of advanced prostate cancer: Results of a randomized multicenter trial. The Prostate. 1991;**18**:139-146

[144] Royer P, Jones K. Progestins for contraception: Modern delivery systems and novel formulations. Clinical Obstetrics and Gynecology. 2014;**57**(4):644-658

[145] Mommers E, Blum G, Gent T, Peters K, Sordal T, Marintcheva-Petrova M. Nexplanon, a radiopaque etonogestrel implant in combination with a next-generation applicator: 3-year results of a noncomparative multicenter trial. American Journal of Obstetrics and Gynecology. 2012;**207**(5): 388.e1-388.e6

[146] Intarcia. n.d. Available from: https://www.intarcia.com/media.html

[147] Rohloff C, Alessi T, Yang B, Dahms J, Carr J, Lautenbach S. DUROS ® technology delivers peptides and proteins at consistent rate continuously for 3 to 12 months. Journal of Diabetes Science and Technology. 2008;**2**(3):461-467

[148] Barrett S, Teller R, Forster S, Li L, Mackey M, Skomski D, et al. Extended-duration MK-8591-eluting implant as a candidate for HIV treatment and prevention. Antimicrobial Agents and Chemotherapy. 2018;**62**:1058-1076

[149] Zaki M, Patil S, Baviskar D, Jain D. Implantable drug delivery system: A review. International Journal of Pharm Tech Research. 2012;**4**(1):280-292

[150] Hu L, Zhang H, Song W. An overview of preparation and evaluation sustained-release injectable microspheres. Journal of Microencapsulation. 2013;**30**(4):369-382

[151] Park E, Amatya S, Kim M, Park J, Seol E, Lee H, et al. Long-acting injectable formulations of antipsychotic drugs for the treatment of schizophrenia. Archives of Pharmacal Research. 2013;**36**(6):651-659

[152] Hoffman A. Hydrogels for biomedical applications. Advanced Drug Delivery Reviews. 2012;**64**:18-23

[153] Kempe S, Mäder K. In situ forming implants—An attractive formulation principle for parenteral depot formulations. Journal of Controlled Release. 2012;**161**(2):668-679

[154] Flexner C. Antiretroviral implants for treatment and prevention of HIV infection. Current Opinion in HIV and AIDS. 2018;**13**(4):374-380

[155] Ruel-Gariépy E, Leroux J. In situ-forming hydrogels—Review of temperature-sensitive systems. European Journal of Pharmaceutics and Biopharmaceutics. 2004;**58**(2):409-426

[156] Available from: https://www.fda.gov/advisory-committees/blood-vaccines-and-other-biologics/cellular-tissue-and-gene-therapies-advisory-committee [Accessed: 28 November 2019]

[157] Fliervoet LAL, Mastrobattista E. Drug delivery with living cells. Advanced Drug Delivery Reviews. 2016;**106**(part A):63-72

[158] O'Brien FJ. Biomaterials & scaffolds for tissue engineering. Materials Today. 2011;**14**(3):88-95

[159] Atala A. Tissue engineering and regenerative medicine: Concepts for clinical application. In: Rejuvenation

Research. Vol. 7. Mary Ann Liebert Inc.; 2004. pp. 15-31

[160] Chen E, Yang L, Ye C, Zhang W, Ran J, Xue D, et al. An asymmetric chitosan scaffold for tendon tissue engineering: In vitro and in vivo evaluation with rat tendon stem/progenitor cells. Acta Biomaterialia. 2018;**73**:377-387

[161] Hazeri Y, Irani S, Zandi M, Pezeshki-Modaress M. Polyvinyl alcohol/sulfated alginate nanofibers induced the neuronal differentiation of human bone marrow stem cells. International Journal of Biological Macromolecules. 2019;**147**:946-953

[162] Kannaiyan J, Khare S, Narayanan S, Mahuvawalla F. Fabrication of electrospun polycaprolactone/gelatin composite nanofibrous scaffolds with cellular responses. American Journal of Nano Research and Applications. 2019;**7**(2):11

[163] Xu F, Ren H, Zheng M, Shao X, Dai T, Wu Y, et al. Development of biodegradable bioactive glass ceramics by DLP printed containing EPCs/BMSCs for bone tissue engineering of rabbit mandible defects. Journal of the Mechanical Behavior of Biomedical Materials. 2020;**103**:103532

[164] Wang H, Shang Y, Cheng X, Wang Z, Zhu D, Liu Y, et al. Delivery of MSCs with a hybrid β-sheet peptide hydrogel consisting IGF-1C domain and D-form peptide for acute kidney injury therapy. SSRN Electronic Journal; 2019;**39**. DOI: 10.2139/ssrn.3485132 [Epub ahead of print]

[165] Gong Z, Lei D, Yu C, Wang C, Xia K, Shu J, et al. Fast degrading bioactive elastic scaffold loaded with neural stem cells promote rapid spinal cord regeneration. SSRN Electronic Journal. 2019. [Epub ahead of print]

[166] Ryu W-S. Diagnosis and methods. In: Molecular Virology of Human Pathogenic Viruses. Cambridge, UK: Elsevier; 2017. pp. 47-62

[167] Buttery LDK, Bishop AE. Introduction to tissue engineering. In: Biomaterials, Artificial Organs and Tissue Engineering. Cambridge, UK: Elsevier Inc.; 2005. pp. 193-200

[168] Kengla C, Kidiyoor A, Murphy SV. Bioprinting complex 3D tissue and organs. In: Kidney Transplantation, Bioengineering, and Regeneration: Kidney Transplantation in the Regenerative Medicine Era. Cambridge, UK: Elsevier Inc.; 2017. pp. 957-971

[169] Rippon HJ, Bishop AE. Embryonic stem cells. Cell Proliferation in Basic and Clinical Sciences. Feb 2004;**37**(1):23-34

[170] Seo BJ, Hong YJ, Do JT. Cellular reprogramming using protein and cell-penetrating peptides [Internet]. International Journal of Molecular Sciences. 2017;**18**:552

[171] Carpenedo RL, McDevitt TC. Stem Cells: Key Concepts. In: Biomaterials Science: An Introduction to Materials. 3rd ed. Cambridge, UK: Elsevier Inc.; 2013. pp. 487-495

[172] Ahmed ASI, Sheng MH, Wasnik S, Baylink DJ, Lau K-HW. Effect of aging on stem cells. World Journal of Experimental Medicine. 2017;**7**(1):1

[173] Beyer Nardi N, Da Silva Meirelles L. Mesenchymal stem cells: Isolation, in vitro expansion and characterization. Handbook of Experimental Pharmacology. 2006;**174**:249-282

[174] Los MJ, Skubis A, Ghavami S. Stem cells. In: Stem Cells and Biomaterials for Regenerative Medicine. Cambridge, UK: Elsevier; 2019. pp. 5-16

[175] Atala A, Lanza R, Thomson JA, Nerem RM. Principles of Regenerative Medicine. Cambridge, UK: Academic Press (Elsevier); 2018. p. 1454

[176] Takahashi K, Yamanaka S. Induction of pluripotent stem cells from mouse embryonic and adult fibroblast cultures by defined factors. Cell. 2006;**126**(4):663-676

[177] Okita K, Ichisaka T, Yamanaka S. Generation of germline-competent induced pluripotent stem cells. Nature. 2007;**448**(7151):313-317

[178] Liu Q, Wang J, Chen Y, Zhang Z, Saunders L, Schipani E, et al. Suppressing mesenchymal stem cell hypertrophy and endochondral ossification in 3D cartilage regeneration with nanofibrous poly(L-lactic acid) scaffold and matrilin-3. Acta Biomaterialia. 2018;**76**:29-38

[179] Salerno A, Fernández-Gutiérrez M, San Román Del Barrio J, Domingo C. Bio-safe fabrication of PLA scaffolds for bone tissue engineering by combining phase separation, porogen leaching and scCO2 drying. Journal of Supercritical Fluids. 2015;**97**:238-246

[180] Fereshteh Z, Fathi M, Bagri A, Boccaccini AR. Preparation and characterization of aligned porous PCL/zein scaffolds as drug delivery systems via improved unidirectional freeze-drying method. Materials Science and Engineering: C. 2016;**68**:613-622

[181] Lowe CJ, Reucroft IM, Grota MC, Shreiber DI. Production of highly aligned collagen scaffolds by freeze-drying of self-assembled, fibrillar collagen gels. ACS Biomaterials Science & Engineering. 2016;**2**(4):643-651

[182] Vishwanath V, Pramanik K, Biswas A. Optimization and evaluation of silk fibroin-chitosan freeze-dried porous scaffolds for cartilage tissue engineering application. Journal of Biomaterials Science, Polymer Edition. 2016;**27**(7):657-674

[183] Li X, Huang L, Li L, Tang Y, Liu Q, Xie H, et al. Biomimetic dual-oriented/bilayered electrospun scaffold for vascular tissue engineering. Journal of Biomaterials Science. Polymer Edition. 2020;**31**(4):1-15

[184] Elizabeth N, Carolina RR, Gowsihan P, Joshua PC, Qun J, Akiko O, et al. Electrospinning 3D bioactive glasses for wound healing. Journal of Biomedical Materials Research. 2020;**15**:015014

[185] Dang W, Ma B, Li B, Huan Z, Ma N, Zhu H, et al. 3D printing of metal-organic framework nanosheets-structured scaffolds with tumor therapy and bone construction. Biofabrication. 2019;**12**(2):025005

[186] Yang Y, Qiao X, Huang R, Chen H, Shi X, Wang J, et al. E-jet 3D printed drug delivery implants to inhibit growth and metastasis of orthotopic breast cancer. Biomaterials. 2019;**13**:119618

[187] Sola A, Bertacchini J, D'Avella D, Anselmi L, Maraldi T, Marmiroli S, et al. Development of solvent-casting particulate leaching (SCPL) polymer scaffolds as improved three-dimensional supports to mimic the bone marrow niche. Materials Science and Engineering: C. 2019;**96**:153-165

[188] Prasad A, Sankar MR, Katiyar V. State of art on solvent casting particulate leaching method for orthopedic scaffoldsfabrication. In: Materials Today: Proceedings. Cambridge, UK: Elsevier Ltd; 2017. pp. 898-907

[189] Yadegari A, Fahimipour F, Rasoulianboroujeni M, Dashtimoghadarm E, Omidi M, Golzar H, et al. Specific considerations in scaffold design for oral tissue engineering. In: Biomaterials for Oral and Dental Tissue Engineering

[Internet]. Cambridge, UK: Woodhead Publishing; 2017. pp. 157-183

[190] Cannillo V, Chiellini F, Fabbri P, Sola A. Production of Bioglass® 45S5—Polycaprolactone composite scaffolds via salt-leaching. Composite Structures. 2010;**92**(8):1823-1832

[191] Eberli D. Tissue Engineering [Internet]. InTech; 2010. p. 536. Available from: http://www.intechopen.com/books/tissue-engineering

[192] Mikos AG, Lu L, Temenoff JS, Tessmar JK. Synthetic bioresorbable polymer scaffolds. In: Biomaterials Science: An Introduction to Materials in Medicine. 2nd ed. Cambridge, UK: Academic Press; 2004. pp. 735-753

[193] Pang WQ, Xu Y. Synthesis and purification at low temperatures. In: Modern Inorganic Synthetic Chemistry. 2nd ed. Cambridge, UK: Elsevier Inc.; 2017. pp. 45-71

[194] Walker JL, Santoro M. Processing and production of bioresorbable polymer scaffolds for tissue engineering. In: Bioresorbable Polymers for Biomedical Applications: From Fundamentals to Translational Medicine. Cambridge, UK: Elsevier; 2016. pp. 181-203

[195] Wahid F, Khan T, Hussain Z, Ullah H. Nanocomposite scaffolds for tissue engineering; properties, preparation and applications. In: Applications of Nanocomposite Materials in Drug Delivery. Cambridge, UK: Elsevier; 2018. pp. 701-735

[196] Girth D, Webster TJ. Matrices for tissue engineering and regenerative medicine [Internet]. Biomaterials for Artificial Organs. Chapter 10. Cambridge, UK: Woodhead Publishing; 2011:270-286

[197] Zafar M, Najeeb S, Khurshid Z, Vazirzadeh M, Zohaib S, Najeeb B, et al. Potential of electrospun nanofibers for biomedical and dental applications. In: Materials. Vol. 9. Basel, Switzerland: MDPI AG; 2016

[198] Hutmacher DW, Woodfield TBF, Dalton PD. Scaffold design and fabrication. In: Tissue Engineering. 2nd ed. Cambridge, UK: Elsevier Inc.; 2014. pp. 311-346

[199] Ma PX, Elisseeff J. Scaffolding in tissue engineering. In: Scaffolding in Tissue Engineering. Boca Raton, FL, USA: CRC Press; 2005. pp. 1-639

[200] Liu J, Yan C. 3D printing of scaffolds for tissue engineering. In: 3D Printing [Internet]. Rijeka: IntechOpen; 2018. Available from: http://www.intechopen.com/books/3d-printing/3d-printing-of-scaffolds-for-tissue-engineering

[201] Billiet T, Vandenhaute M, Schelfhout J, Van Vlierberghe S, Dubruel P. A review of trends and limitations in hydrogel-rapid prototyping for tissue engineering. Biomaterials. 2012;**33**:6020-6041

[202] Skoog SA, Goering PL, Narayan RJ. Stereolithography in tissue engineering. Journal of Materials Science: Materials in Medicine. 2014;**25**:845-856

[203] Kumar S. Selective laser sintering: A qualitative and objective approach. Journal of Minerals, Metals and Materials Society. 2003;**55**(10):43-47

[204] Ambrosi A, Pumera M. 3D-printing technologies for electrochemical applications. Chemical Society Reviews and Royal Society of Chemistry. 2016;**45**(10):2740-2755

[205] Yan X, Gu P. A review of rapid prototyping technologies and systems. In: CAD Computer Aided Design. Vol. 28. Cambridge, UK: Elsevier Ltd; 1996. pp. 307-318

[206] Masood SH. Advances in fused deposition modeling. In: Comprehensive

Materials Processing. Cambridge, UK: Elsevier Ltd; 2014. pp. 69-91

[207] Dayan CB, Afghah F, Okan BS, Yıldız M, Menceloglu Y, Culha M, et al. Modeling 3D melt electrospinning writing by response surface methodology. Materials and Design. 2018;**148**:87-95

[208] Tourlomousis F, Ding H, Kalyon DM, Chang RC. Melt electrospinning writing process guided by a "Printability Number". Journal of Manufacturing Science and Engineering, Transactions of the ASME. 2017;**139**(8):081004-1 to 081004-15

[209] Do A-V, Smith R, Acri TM, Geary SM, Salem AK. 3D printing technologies for 3D scaffold engineering. In: Deng Y, Kuiper J, editors. Functional 3D Tissue Engineering Scaffolds. Cambridge, UK: Elsevier; 2018. pp. 203-234

[210] Taboas JM, Maddox RD, Krebsbach PH, Hollister SJ. Indirect solid free form fabrication of local and global porous, biomimetic and composite 3D polymer-ceramic scaffolds. Biomaterials. 2003;**24**(1):181-194

[211] Hernández-Córdova R, Mathew DA, Balint R, Carrillo-Escalante HJ, Cervantes-Uc JM, Hidalgo-Bastida LA, et al. Indirect three-dimensional printing: A method for fabricating polyurethane-urea based cardiac scaffolds. Journal of Biomedical Materials Research Part A. 2016;**104**(8):1912-1921

[212] Ebnesajjad S. Injection molding. Fluoroplastics. 2015;2:236-281

[213] Huang B, Liang S, Qu X. The rheology of metal injection molding. Journal of Materials Processing Technology. 2003;**137**(1-3):132-137

[214] Ghalia MA, Dahman Y. Advanced nanobiomaterials in tissue engineering: Synthesis, properties, and applications. In: Nanobiomaterials in Soft Tissue Engineering: Applications of Nanobiomaterials. Cambridge, UK: Elsevier Inc.; 2016. pp. 141-172

[215] Habibi N, Kamaly N, Memic A, Shafiee H. Self-assembled peptide-based nanostructures: Smart nanomaterials toward targeted drug delivery. Nano Today. Elsevier B.V. 2016;**11**(1):41-60

[216] Greenbaum J. Regulation of drug–device combination products in the USA. In: Greenbaum J, Lewis A, editors. Drug-Device Combination Products. 1st ed. Cambridge, UK: Woodhead Publishing; 2010. pp. 496-529

[217] Leppard S. Regulation of drug–device combination products in Europe. In: Leppard S, Lewis A, editors. Drug-Device Combination Products. 1st ed. Cambridge, UK: Woodhead Publishing.; 2010. pp. 464-495

[218] Ratner B, Hoffman A, Schoen F, Lemons J, editors. Voluntary standards, regulatory compliance, and non-technical issues. In: Biomaterials Science. 3rd ed. Cambridge, UK: Elsevier; 2012. pp. 1387-1472

[219] Ragelle H, Danhier F, Préat V, Langer R, Anderson D. Nanoparticle-based drug delivery systems: A commercial and regulatory outlook as the field matures. Expert Opinion on Drug Delivery. 2017;**14**(7):851-864

[220] Lambert B, Martin J. Sterilization of implants and devices. In: Lambert B, Martin J, Ratner B, Hoffman A, Schoen F, Lemons J, editors. Biomaterials Science. 3rd ed. London, UK: Elsevier; 2013. pp. 1339-1353

Chapter 2

Dental Implants

İhsan Çağlar Çınar, B. Alper Gültekin, Alper Sağlanmak and Cem Töre

Abstract

The goal of modern dentistry is to return patients to oral health in a predictable fashion. The partial and complete edentulous patient may be unable to recover normal function, esthetics, comfort, or speech with a traditional removable prosthesis. The patient's function when wearing a denture may be reduced to one sixth of the level formerly experienced with natural dentition; however, an implant prosthesis may return the function to near-normal limits. The esthetics of the edentulous patient is affected as a result of muscle and bone atrophy. In order to replace a missing tooth, the development of materials science and technology improved the materials for implant application. Nowadays, titanium has become the most popular implant material due to its advantages. The first submerged implant placed by Strock was still functioning 40 years later. Recently, zirconia implants and innovative surface designs are being researched and practiced. In this chapter, these materials will be comparatively discussed through contemporary literature and research.

Keywords: implant corrosion, dental implants, oral implantology, titanium implants, zirconia implants, oxide layer, zirconium dioxide, Ti-6Al-4V, calcium phosphate ceramics, osseointegration

1. Introduction

Modern dentistry aims to restore a patient's oral esthetics, contour, function, and speech. Depending on the patient's needs, the total treatment may range from treating a single tooth with caries to restoring edentulous arches with severe bone resorption.

Implant dentistry has made predictable success a reality for cases in the more difficult part of this spectrum through research, improvements in diagnostic tools, techniques, implant materials, and designs. Endosteal implants are manufactured materials inserted in edentulous ridges via surgery so they can serve as a foundation for the prosthesis [1]. Most implants that will be discussed in this chapter will be root form implants which mimic the root shape of a tooth.

1.1 History of dental implants

The desire to restore lost teeth is not a new concept. Dental implant surgery is one of the oldest practices in dentistry second only to tooth extractions. There is archeological evidence that humans have attempted to replace missing teeth with root form implants for thousands of years. Remains from ancient China dating

4000 years ago have carved bamboo pegs, tapped into the bone, to replace lost teeth, and 2000-year-old remains from ancient Egypt have similarly shaped pegs made of precious metals. Some Egyptian mummies were found to have transplanted human teeth, and in other instances, teeth made of ivory [2]. Central American Incas tapped seashells in bone similar to the Chinese [3].

In 1809, Maggiolo introduced root shaped gold implants followed by Harris introducing porcelain teeth supported by lead-coated platinum posts [4, 5]. Gold, magnesium, copper, brass, aluminum, silver, and soft steel plated with nickel and gold was used to fabricate implants by Lambotte in 1900s [6]. Corrosion of most of these metals by body tissues was observed which in return caused electrolytic action. In 1909, Greenfield introduced an implant in the form of a cylindrical lattice-cage which differed substantially from the root form implants [7]. A calibrated cylindrical bur was used for the osteotomy to preserve an inner core of bone within the implant. This was also the first design which separated the endosteal implant from the abutment which was to be connected on the implant weeks later through an internal attachment after healing. In 1940, Bothe described a titanium implant and bone interface as bone fusing [8]. The first two-piece titanium screw-type implant was designed in 1946 by Strock [9]. The direct implant-bone interface desired by Strock was called ankylosis.

Brånemark's studies in bone marrow healing in 1952 led to dental implant application in dogs in early 1960s, and implant integrations in bone were achieved without adverse reaction in surrounding tissues. Implant applications in humans with Brånemark philosophy were started in 1965, and 10-year results were published in 1977 [10]. Osseointegration, which has become the term used today for implants instead of ankylosis or bone fusing, was defined by Brånemark as a direct contact between the implant surface and living bone that can be observed through a light microscope [11].

Through advances in material sciences, manufacturing processes, research, and clinical studies, the usage of dental implants have become an essential part of contemporary restorative dentistry.

1.2 Dental implant material properties

1.2.1 Metals and alloys

Majority of the dental implants to date have been fabricated from metals and alloys. American Society for Testing and Materials and International Standards Organization have created guidelines for standardizing implant materials [12, 13].

1.2.1.1 Titanium and titanium: 6 aluminum: 4 vanadium (Ti-6Al-4V)

Titanium and its alloys are the most widely used materials for dental implants [14]. This metal group forms retentive oxides in contact with room temperature air or solutions containing oxygen such as tissue fluids. This provides an advantage since this titanium oxide surface minimizes biocorrosion. In the case of an oxide surface becoming scratched or removed during implant placement into bone, the surface reoxidizes in the bone tissue. This regenerative biocorrosion preventing layer is one of the reasons for the wide use of titanium in dental implants [15].

Bothe et al. reported bone growth in contact with titanium surfaces in rabbits [8]. Several researchers studied and expanded the indications for use of titanium in implant devices. The reason reported is titanium's non-reactive nature and its resilience to corrosion [16, 17]. General properties of alloys and metal used in implant fabrication are detailed in **Table 1** [12].

	Nominal analysis (w/o)	Modulus of elasticity GN/m² (psi µ 10⁶)	Ultimate tensile strength MN/m² (ksi)	Elongation to fracture (%)
Titanium	99+Ti	97 (14)	240–550 (25–70)	>15
Titanium-aluminum-vanadium	90Ti-6Al-4V	117 (17)	869–896 (125–130)	>12
Cobalt-chromium-molybdenum (casting)	66Co-27Cr-7Mo	235 (34)	655 (95)	>8
Stainless steel (316 L)	70Fe-18Cr-12Ni	193 (28)	480–1000 (70–145)	>30
Zirconium	99+Zr	97 (14)	552 (80)	20
Tantalum	99+Ta	—	690 (100)	11
Gold	99+Au	97 (14)	207–310 (30–45)	>30
Platinum	99+Pt	166 (24)	131 (19)	40

Table 1.
Mechanical properties of various alloys and metals used in implants [13, 14].

The titanium alloy with the most widespread use is titanium-aluminum-vanadium. This alloy has approximately six times the strength of compact bone, and as a result, thinner structural parts can be incorporated into the implants without risking breakage or cracking. The alloys modulus of elasticity is 5.6 times greater than compact bone. Several studies have investigated and documented the titanium oxide layer on both pure titanium and its alloy which can vary depending on surface properties [18]. The techniques for casting titanium and alloys are limited because of high melting points and high chance of hydrogen, nitrogen, and oxygen absorption. Different purity levels can be achieved through an ultrapure protective gas environment or a high vacuum [18].

1.2.1.2 Cobalt-chromium-molybdenum-based alloy

This alloy is made up of cobalt, chromium, and molybdenum. Alloys containing cobalt are usually used as they are cast and are sometimes additionally annealed. This allows custom designs otherwise unachievable. The named elements with minor additions of nickel, manganese, and carbon provide strength four times greater than compact bone and chromium provides resistance to corrosion. These concentrations are critical so the fabrication processes must be carefully controlled and followed. Cobalt-based alloys are the least ductile of the ones used in dental implants [12]. Excellent biocompatibility has been observed with implants from cobalt-based alloys when they are manufactured properly.

1.2.1.3 Iron-chromium-nickel-based alloys

Stainless steel alloys are one of the oldest materials to be used in the medical field. The alloy is most often used in a wrought and heat treated condition, same as titanium alloys, which gives the material high strength and ductility. Among all alloys used in implant fabrication steel alloys are the ones most susceptible to biocorrosion so the applied oxide surface must be protected. Another concerning aspect of iron-based alloys are galvanic potentials. If a steel-based implant abutment contacted a bridge containing a noble metal, for example, a circuit would be formed. This would not be a cause of concern if these units function without contact [19, 20].

1.2.1.4 Other metals and alloys

Several other metals been used in implant manufacturing. Notably, among these, gold and platinum have been evaluated but the low strength of these materials limit implant design.

1.2.2 Ceramics

Ceramics are non-metal, non-polymer, inorganic materials. Oxide ceramic dental implants were fabricated to make use of their resistance to biodegradation, strength, color, low conductivity, and elastic properties [21, 22]. Despite their low ductility and brittle nature, ceramics are being used both as coatings on other materials and in bulk form.

1.2.2.1 Aluminum, titanium, and zirconium oxides

Main properties of these materials are listed in **Table 2** [12]. High strength oxide ceramics have been used as several implant forms including root form implants [23]. Ceramics have approximately 3–5 times the strength of compact bone. Creating a different implant design for these materials is necessary because of their high strength and high modulus of elasticity. Metallic oxide ceramics generally have a white hue of color which makes them a viable option for implants in the esthetic area in cases where gingival recession leaves implants visible. When compared with other materials, minimal reactivity with oral tissues paired with low electrical and thermal conductivity are notable benefits.

As with titanium implants, bone growth directly adjacent to the implant surface has been observed. Going a step further, areas of bonding have been reported in gingival attachment zones of sapphire dental implants in animal studies [24–26]. There are also special requirements for sterilization of metallic oxide ceramic implants. Since steam and chemical solutions can lead to micro weaknesses which can lead to fractures or leftover residues; dry heat is the best choice for sterilization of ceramics. Their improved strength and excellent biocompatibility make ceramics a viable choice as an implant material.

	Modulus of elasticity GN/m^2 (psi µ 10^6)	**Ultimate bending strength MN/m^2 (ksi)**	**Elongation to fracture (%)**	**Surface**
Polycrystalline aluminum oxide	372 (54)	300–550 (43–80)	0	Al_2O_3
Single crystal aluminum oxide (sapphire)	392 (56)	640 (93)	0	Al_2O_3
Zirconium oxide zirconia (PSZ)	195–210 (28–30)	500–650 (72–94)	0	ZrO_2
Titanium oxide (titania)	280 (41)	69–103 (10–15)	0	TiO_2

Table 2.
Mechanical properties of various inert ceramics [13, 14].

1.2.2.2 Calcium phosphate ceramics (CPC)

First implants manufactured from CPCs aimed to reduce bone resorption after tooth extractions by filling the bone socket with cone-shaped implants [27]. The materials limited strength led researchers to either reinforcing the material internally with metal parts or to coat other materials with CPCs [28]. Out of these techniques, coating metal implants via flame or plasma spraying was more widely used with the intent of making metal implants more biocompatible [29].

The advantages of the application are the materials chemical similarity to living tissues, biocompatibility, and low conductivity which means it can act as a barrier to metallic ion transport between bone and metal implants. Disadvantages are its low strength and the materials possibility to dissolve or alter in time. Main properties of these materials can be found in **Table 3** [12]. Generally, bioceramics are characterized by lower hardness, strength, and elasticity modulus than ceramics like zirconia or aluminum oxide. Overall, CPCs are one of the most widely accepted, studied, and used biomaterials developed in the last decades and could find its applications expanding further as future implant surfaces as they evolve themselves through technology and research [30].

1.2.2.3 Carbon and carbon silicon compounds

Carbon and carbon silicon materials are regarded as ceramics for their non-reactive nature, but they conduct electricity and heat. Its elasticity is close to bone, and it is a biocompatible material. Clinical trials of carbon-based dental implants were carried out. Limitations in material properties, design, and applications led to clinical failures in trials which resulted in withdrawal of carbon-based materials in dental implant designs.

1.3 Influence of dental implant materials on soft and hard tissue

1.3.1 Implant surgery

Implant surgery begins with an incision on the edentulous ridge and flap elevation to expose the alveolar bone. At the end of the surgery, the same flap will be sutured and a primary wound healing of masticatory mucosa will follow. If a submerged (placed under oral mucosa level) implant is being used, a recovery surgery will be performed after a period of healing. If a non-submerged (placed on the same level as oral mucosa) implant is being used, no recovery surgery is necessary.

	Modulus of elasticity GN/m^2 (psi μ 10^6)	Ultimate bending strength MN/m^2 (ksi)	Elongation to fracture (%)	Surface
Hydroxyapatite	40–120 (6–17)	40–300 (6–43)	0	$Ca_{10}(PO_4)_6(OH)_2$
Tricalcium phosphate	30–120 (4–17)	15–120 (2–17)	0	$Ca_3(PO_4)_2$
Bioglass or Ceravital	40–140 (6–20)	20–350 (3–51)	0	$CaPO_4$
Carbon	25–40 (4–6)	150–250 (22–36)	0	C
Carbon-silicon (LTI)	25–40 (4–6)	200–700 (29–101)	0	CSi

Table 3.
Mechanical properties of various bioactive ceramics [13, 14].

Most implant systems available today allow creation of a recipient intrabony site for implant placement via rotary instruments. A tight fit is crucial for primary stabilization of the implant and for preventing soft tissue from penetrating the gap between the implant and the bone, effectively preventing the implant osseointegration.

Most important negative influence of the surgery stage can be creation of excessive heat with rotary instruments. It has been shown that bringing of the temperature of bone to 47°C for 1 minute is enough to kill osteogenic cells which can compromise necessary healing. As a safety measure, several sharp drills must be used at low speeds with low hand pressure and proper irrigation for cooling the site [31].

1.3.2 Long-term influences on peri-implant tissues

Following surgery if no infection or inflammatory response takes place to prevent healing, primary wound healing defines the long-term properties of surrounding tissues. Regardless of the dental implant material, the general outcome of bone healing around an implant is osseointegration which is defined by Brånemark as "a direct structural and functional connection between ordered, living bone and the surface of a load-carrying implant [11]." Throughout several weeks of healing, woven bone which forms during early stages of healing starts to become more compact lamellar bone. This formation can be observed both from the cut bone and from the implant surface [32].

Titanium's corrosion rate in tissues is well documented [33]. In older studies, the presence of titanium has been detected in peri-implant tissues and internal organs, presumed to be caused by corrosion, mechanical wear, and peri-implant inflammation, but the compositions of the implant alloys were not strictly controlled, and in same studies, the diffusion is very slow and since titanium has little to no toxicity, it should be considered biocompatible [34, 35]. In a recent study, titanium particles have been detected in healthy and inflamed mucosa and even in patients with no titanium implants [36]. The increased amount of particles is likely the effect of the inflammation rather than its cause. Since then, higher strength alloys of titanium have emerged [37]. Recently, applications of these materials have been successful and have not resulted in significant negative effects. Titanium allergy has been studied and is known to be rare, but research is insufficient to give an accurate incidence rate [38].

The oxide surface of titanium as previously discussed exists through reacting with oxygen at normal temperatures and will rapidly reform if removed mechanically. It minimizes biocorrosion in tissues [15]. The oxide layer consists of mostly TiO_2 and to a lesser degree Ti_2O_3 and TiO [39]. While in normal temperatures, the oxide layer is less than 20 nm in thickness, when processed at high temperatures or anodized at high voltages, the layer can be 10–100 times thicker in a crystalline structure [40]. The macro and micro architecture of dental implants achieved via sand blasting, acid etching, or mechanical milling has no significant effect over the thickness of the oxide layer [41]. Naturally occurring oxidants in tissues such as hydrogen peroxide has been shown to form a complex gel with titanium on a molecular level. This layer is found to have a very low toxicity, anti-inflammatory, and bactericidal properties [42].

Coating titanium implants by hydroxyapatite via plasma spraying is a method developed to help minimize ion transfer and accelerate bone formation between the bone-implant interface [43]. The disadvantages of this coating are its possibility of partial resorption during bone remodeling, after in vivo function, or in inflammation areas [44]. A recent study tested titanium and cobalt implants coated with zirconium nitride and found the product to be cytocompatible and the red color range can potentially minimize the visibility of implants under the gingiva [45].

Aluminum oxide ceramics are used as implant bulk materials one advantage is having the oxide layer properties throughout the entire body of the implant. As a result, any removal of surface has no effect on the electrochemical properties underneath the surface. Ceramic coatings aim to give the same biocompatibility advantages to metals or alloys to be coated [46]. A systematic review including six randomized controlled trials (RCTs) studied implants consisting of 85% Ti and 15% Zr found that narrow Ti-Zr implants have comparable performance to regular diameter Ti implants noting further research is necessary [47]. Some studies tested alloys consisting of Ti-Nb and found the material to be cytocompatible and a good candidate for implantology in future research due to its very low elasticity modulus [48, 49].

1.4 Success of dental implant materials

There have been different criteria for measuring success of dental implants. The two most commonly used in literature is survival and success. Survival of an implant states whether the implant is simply still functioning in the mouth or it has been removed. Success on the other hand is concerned with the condition of peri-implant tissues and teeth as well as patients comfort and satisfaction [50].

A systematic review evaluating 23 published articles and 7711 implants over a minimum of 10 and a mean of 13.4 years found a survival rate of 94.6% and a mean bone loss of 1.3 mm around implants [51].

An article on zirconia dental implants stated zirconium dioxide is a promising alternative for titanium, but studies found significantly more early failures compared to titanium. Technical advances and innovation are found to be promising; however, there is insufficient evidence for a final verdict at present [52]. An ITI consensus report from 2018 states one-piece zirconia implants are safe in appropriate conditions but cautions against two-piece zirconia implants due to insufficient data. Same report stated that throughout different implant loading protocols and implant materials, survival rates are above 96% [53]. A meta-analysis evaluating 17 studies reviewing clinical outcomes of zirconium dioxide implants states that the survival rate was 95% over 1–7 years of follow-up [54]. A study on properties of porous tantalum found the materials similarity to bone in terms of mechanical properties and that it has less cytotoxicity than titanium. The authors claim bone growth into the implant surface to form a unique interface pattern but state tantalums safety and performance as an implant material should be further tested [55].

The lack of long-term follow-ups for zirconia implants result in researchers advising caution and stating the information in insufficient even when high survival rates are found and zirconium dioxide implants are becoming a viable alternative to metal implants.

Titanium implants in contrast have very well-documented success with follow-ups exceeding 25 years [56]. The current research in titanium implants is not concerned of success of the material but rather its viability and applications in diabetics, smokers, patients who underwent radiotherapy or anti-resorptive drugs as well as timing of implantation and loading.

1.5 Potential impacts of titanium

Titanium and its alloys have been widely and safely used in the field of oral implantology for 40 years. In the early years, researchers have argued that titanium is a bio-inert material, but with recent studies, it has been found that titanium degradation, as particle or ion release may penetrate surrounding tissues. This degradation can occur during implantation, during the prosthesis stage, or many years after loading, during maintenance. The surface of an implant is covered with many atomic-sized titanium oxide layers for its benefit in osseointegration and corrosion resistance. Degradation of this layer over time may cause ion release from the implant surface. The compressive and frictional forces generated during osteotomy in surgical phase may disrupt this structure and cause titanium particle release. It is also possible that the biofilm formed in the abutment-implant connection, which is the weakest component of an implant, acts as a lubricant, and thus results in micro-movement and wear on the inner surface of the implant. Finally, with the exposure of the implant surface during maintenance, chemical changes may occur on the surface of the implant with factors such as saliva and bacteria. Cleaning of implants surface with various instruments may also cause titanium release [57]. Titanium release, which may occur due to the reasons listed above, has been held responsible for peri-implant diseases such as mucositis and periimplantitis in recent years. Oliviera et al. reported that titanium particles increase osteoclast activity and cause mutational changes in cells. As a result, it was argued that titanium release from the implant surface is responsible for peri-implant tissue destruction with its cytotoxic and genotoxic effect [58]. In many studies, titanium nanoparticles phagocytosed by macrophages were found in histological examination of specimens taken from the surrounding infected tissue. In a study by Wennerberg et al., implants with moderately rough surfaces emit much more titanium than other implant surfaces. The same study argues that the titanium oxide layer oscillates more easily in additive surfaces than the surfaces formed by subtraction [59]. In the light of all this information, it is not possible to say that titanium used in dental implant applications is bio-inert. Due to the surface structure of the implant, bone density, overloading, and various many different factors, potential influences in degradation of the implant surface come in sight and harmful effects on the surrounding tissues can occur [60]. On the other hand, the peripheral organ impacts of titanium are still controversial. Although it is not possible to completely eliminate the titanium particle release, there are some ways to minimize titanium release. Today, the use of different materials that are more resistant to abrasion (such as zirconium, tantalium, etc.) has come to the fore in order to protect against the possible harmful effects of titanium.

1.5.1 Implant macrogeometry

Implant macrogeometry, which can also be defined as implant design, has been one of the most researched topics in recent years. However, before examining thoroughly into this topic, it is necessary to know the two popular hypotheses that implant success and survival are based on. The first one is the "Biological Hypothesis" which declares, marginal bone loss mostly depends on bacterial plaque and the host response. "Biomechanical Hypothesis," which became a current factor, advocates the effect of occlusal excessive forces on the bone surrounding implants and compression, tension, and shear forces during and after osseointegration are crucial in implant survival and success. According to the biomechanical hypothesis, implant design is the key that provides primary stability of the implant and resistance of the implant to forces during and after osseointegration. Primary and secondary osseointegration degrees and durations of the implant have been correlated with macrogeometry in many studies. The reason for this fact is that implant macrogeometry affects the host-implant response [61]. According to these studies, the healing time of implants was shortened with the development of implant macrogeometries, and the possibility of immediate or early loading of implants came to the fore. Especially in recent years within the scope of macrogeometry, many studies have been examining implant abutment connection, implant neck design, and their effects on long-term preservation of crestal bone. Nowadays, the aim should be to achieve an ideal implant macrogeometry to put the implants into function in the shortest time and to ensure their long-term function. The body shape, groove design, or groove geometry (groove shape, groove spacing, groove depth, groove width, implant groove surface angle, and helix angle), prosthetic interface, and implant neck design forms the macrogeometry of an implant.

1.5.2 Implant microgeometry

The concept of implant microgeometry was first described by Geng et al. in 2004 consists of implant surface topography, implant surface coating, and implant material [62]. In addition, Albrektsson et al. identified six factors for reliable osseointegration. Surface quality is one of the six factors that plays a key role in the host's response to the implant.

1.5.2.1 Implant surface topography and implant surface coating

The term implant surface refers to an outer layer of 1–2 nm which includes several outermost atomic layers different from the body material. This outermost layer is seen as the thickness of the titanium oxide layer and the structure that can be responsible for the reactions that occur on the surface. Implant surface modification can be performed in two ways by forming concave or convex surface tissue. Various methods such as sandblasting, turning, chemical and electrochemical pickling, laser application, and anodizing are used for roughening of surfaces. The amount of roughness of the resulting surface can range from nanometers to millimeters [63]. A number of studies have shown that rough surface implants have a stronger connection with bone; this structure stops the migration of epithelial attachment to the apical, thus preventing crestal bone resorption [64].

2. Conclusion

The discipline of oral implantology has come a long way from its state in 1960s. This is largely due to the rapid evolution of biomaterials discipline in 1970s. With new biomaterials and advances in surgical techniques, dental implantology is a highly successful field, consistently publishing articles reporting success rates of 90% and above over long follow-ups. Biomaterials are now manufactured and provided as sterile, standardized devices with high predictability which is essential in the field of medicine. This requirement of predictability is the reason titanium implants with widely used, well-documented surface properties are the gold standard and are the most common biomaterial of choice in dental implant devices. In recent years, zirconium implants have been rising in popularity and dependable short-term clinical outcomes look promising, but future research of long-term clinical outcomes is necessary to safely recommend and expand the indications of zirconia implants.

Conflict of interest

The authors declare no conflict of interest.

Author details

İhsan Çağlar Çınar, B. Alper Gültekin*, Alper Sağlanmak and Cem Töre
Istanbul University, Istanbul, Turkey

*Address all correspondence to: alpergultekin@hotmail.com

References

[1] Cranin AN. Glossary of implant terms. The Journal of Oral Implantology. 1990;**16**:57-63

[2] Misch CE. Contemporary Implant Dentistry. St. Louis, Missouri: Mosby Elsevier; 2007

[3] Anjard R. Mayan dental wonders. Oral Implantology. 1981;**9**:423

[4] Maggiolo: Manuel de l'art dentaire [Manual of Dental Art], Nancy, France, C Le Seure; 1809

[5] Harris LM. An artifi cial crown on a leaden root. Dental Cosmos. 1887;**55**:433

[6] Lambotte A. New instruction for the banding of bone: Banding with a screw. J C Ann Soc Belge Chir. 1909;**9**:113

[7] Greenfield EJ. Implantation of artificial crowns and bridge abutments. Dent Cosmos. 1913;**55**:364-430

[8] Bothe RT, Beaton LE, Davenport HA. Reaction of bone to multiple metallic implants. Surgery, Gynecology & Obstetrics. 1940;**71**:598-602

[9] Strock AE, Strock MS. Further Studies on Inert Metal Implantation for Replacement. Alpha Omega; 1949

[10] Brånemark PI, Hansson BO, Adell R, et al. Osseointegrated implants in the treatment of the edentulous jaw: Experience from a 10-year period. Scandinavian Journal of Plastic and Reconstructive Surgery. Supplementum. 1977;**16**:1-132

[11] Brånemark PI. GA Zarb, and T Albrektsson: Tissue Integrated Prostheses. Quintessence, Chicago: Osseointegration in Clinical Dentistry; 1985

[12] American Society for Testing and Materials. Surgical and Medical Devices. Vol. 14.01. Philadelphia: American Society for Testing and Materials; 1996

[13] International Standards Organization. Standard References. Philadelphia: ANSI-USA; 1996

[14] International Standardization Organization. Technical Report 10451: Dental Implants—State of the Art—Survey of Materials. Geneva; 1991

[15] Rae T. The biological response to titanium and titanium aluminum vanadium alloy particles. Biomaterials. 1986;7:3036

[16] Lemons JE, Niemann KMW, Weiss AB. Biocompatibility studies on surgical grade Ti, Co and Fe base alloys. Journal of Biomedical Materials Research. 1976;**10**:549

[17] Lucas LC, Lemons JE, Lee J, et al. In vitro corrosion characteristics of Co-Cr-Mo/Ti-6Al-4V/Ti alloys. In: Paper presented at the American Society for Testing Materials, Symposium on Quantitative Characteristics of Porous Materials for Host Tissues, 1978

[18] Davies JE, editor. The Bone-Biomaterial Interface. Toronto: University of Toronto Press; 1991

[19] Lucas LC, Buchanan RA, Lemons JE. Investigations on the galvanic corrosion of multialloy total hip prostheses. Journal of Biomedical Materials Research. 1981;**15**:731-747

[20] Lucas LC, Buchanan RA, Lemons JE, et al. Susceptibility of surgical cobalt-base alloy to pitting corrosion. Journal of Biomedical Materials Research. 1982;**16**:799-810

[21] Hench LL, Ethridge EC. Biomaterials, an Interfacial Approach. New York: Academic Press; 1982

[22] Vincenzini P, editor. Ceramics in Surgery. Amsterdam: Elsevier; 1983

[23] Sandhaus S. Nouveaux aspects de l'implantologie, L'Implant CBS Suisse. Lausanne, Switzerland: Sandhaus; 1969

[24] Steflic D, Sisk A, Parr G, et al. HVEM and conventional electron microscopy of interface between bone and endosteal dental implants. Journal of Biomedical Materials Research. 1992; **26**:529-545

[25] McKinney R, Steflic DE, Koth D, et al. The scientific basis for dental implant therapy. Journal of Dental Education. 1988;**52**:696-705

[26] Koth DL, McKinney RV Jr. The single crystal sapphire endosteal dental implant. In: Hardin JF, editor. Clark's Clinical Dentistry. Philadelphia: JB Lippincott; 1981

[27] Kent J et al. Augmentation of defi cient edentulous alveolar ridges with dense polycrystalline hydroxylapatite (abstract 3.8.2). In: Final Program and Book of Abstracts. Vienna: First World Biomaterials Congress, Society for Biomaterials; 1980

[28] English C. Cylindrical implants. Journal of the California Dental Association. 1988;**16**:17-40

[29] Ducheyne P, Hench LL, Kagan A, et al. Effect of hydroxyapatite impregnation on skeletal bonding of porous coated implants. Journal of Biomedical Materials Research. 1987;**14**: 225-237

[30] Lemons JE. Ceramics: Past, present and future. Bone. 1996;**19**(suppl):121S-128S

[31] Eriksson AR, Albrektsson T. Temperature threshold levels for heat-induced bone tissue injury: A vital-microscopic study in the rabbit. The Journal of Prosthetic Dentistry. 1983; **50**(1):101-107

[32] Nanci A, McCarthy GF, Zalzal S, Clokie CML, Warshawsky H, McKee MD. Tissue response to titanium implants in the rat tibia: Ultrastructural, immunocytochemical and lectincytochemical characterization of the bone-titanium interface. Cells & Materials. 1994;**4**:1-30

[33] Steinemann SG. Corrosion of titanium and titanium alloys for surgical implants. In: Lutering G, Zwicker U, Bunk W, editors. Proceedings of the 5th International Conference on Titanium, Dtsch Gesf Materialkunde eV. Vol. 2. 1985. pp. 1373-1379

[34] Woodman JL, Jacobs JJ, Galante JO, et al. Metal ion release from titanium-based prosthetic segmental replacement of long bones in baboons. A long-term study. Journal of Orthopaedic Research. 1984;**1**:421-430

[35] Osborn JF, Willich P, Meenen N. The release of titanium into human bone from a titanium implant coated with plasma-sprayed titanium. In: Heimke G, Solesz U, AJC L, editors. Advances in Biomaterials. Amsterdam; 1990

[36] Noumbiss S, Scarano A, Gupta S. A literature review study on atomic ions dissolution of titanium and its alloys in implant dentistry. Materials. 2019;**12**(3): 368

[37] Lemons JE. Metals and alloys for devices in musculoskeletal surgery. In: Morrey BF, editor. Joint Replacement Arthroplasty. Edinburgh: Churchill Livingstone; 1991

[38] Goutam M, Giriyapura C, Mishra SK, Gupta S. Titanium allergy: A literature review. Indian Journal of Dermatology. 2014;**59**(6):630

[39] Lausmaa J, Kasemo B, Mattson H. Surface spectroscopic characterization

of titanium implant materials. Applied Surface Science. 1990;**44**:133-146

[40] Ong JL, Lucas LC, Connatser RW, et al. Spectroscopic characterization of passivated titanium in a physiological solution. Journal of Materials Science. Materials in Medicine. 1995;**6**:113-119

[41] Smith DC, Piliar RM, Chernecky R. Dental implant materials. I. some effects of preparative procedures on surface topography. Journal of Biomedical Materials Research. 1991;**25**: 1045-1068

[42] Tengvall P, Lindstrom I. Physicochemical considerations of titanium as biomaterial. Clinical Materials. 1992;**9**:115-134

[43] Block MS, Kent JN, Kay JF. Evaluation of hydroxylapatitecoated titanium dental implants in dogs. Journal of Oral and Maxillofacial Surgery. 1987;**45**:601-607

[44] Caulier H, Vercaigne S, Naert I, et al. The effect of Ca-P plasma sprayed coatings on the initial bone healing of oral implants and experimental study in the goat. Biomedical Materials Research. 1997;**34**:121-128

[45] Prachar P, Bartakova S, Brezina V, Cvrcek L, Vanek J. Cytocompatibility of implants coated with titanium nitride and zirconium nitride. Bratislava Medical Journal. 2015;**116**(03):154-156

[46] Sella C, Martin JC, Lecoeur J, et al. Biocompatibility and corrosion resistance in biological media of hard ceramic coatings sputter deposited on metal implants. Materials Science & Engineering A: Structural Materials. 1991;**139**:49-57

[47] Badran Z, Struillou X, Strube N, Bourdin D, Dard M, Soueidan A, et al. Clinical performance of narrow-diameter titanium-zirconium implants. Implant Dentistry. 2017;**26**(2):316-323

[48] Fischer M, Laheurte P, Acquier P, Joguet D, Peltier L, Petithory T, et al. Synthesis and characterization of Ti-27.5Nb alloy made by CLAD® additive manufacturing process for biomedical applications. Materials Science and Engineering: C. 2017;**75**:341-348

[49] Fischer M, Joguet D, Robin G, Peltier L, Laheurte P. In situ elaboration of a binary Ti–26Nb alloy by selective laser melting of elemental titanium and niobium mixed powders. Materials Science and Engineering: C. 2016;**62**: 852-859

[50] Council on Scientific Affairs. Dental endosseous implants: An update. Journal of the American Dental Association (1939). 1996;**129**:1238-1239

[51] Moraschini V et al. Evaluation of survival and success rates of dental implants reported in longitudinal studies with a follow-up period of at least 10 years: A systematic review. International Journal of Oral and Maxillofacial Surgery. 2015;**44**(3): 377-388

[52] Cionca N, Hashim D, Mombelli A. Zirconia dental implants: Where are we now, and where are we heading? Periodontology 2000. 2016;**73**(1): 241-258

[53] Morton D et al. Group 2 ITI consensus report: Prosthodontics and implant dentistry. Clinical Oral Implants Research. 2018;**29**:215-223

[54] Haro Adánez M, Nishihara H, Att W. A systematic review and meta-analysis on the clinical outcome of zirconia implant–restoration complex. Journal of Prosthodontic Research. 2018;**62**(4):397-406

[55] Liu Y, Bao C, Wismeijer D, Wu G. The physicochemical/biological properties of porous tantalum and the potential surface modification techniques to improve its clinical

application in dental implantology. Materials Science and Engineering: C. 2015;**49**:323-329

[56] Jemt T. Implant survival in the edentulous jaw—30 years of experience. Part I: A retro-prospective multivariate regression analysis of overall implant failure in 4,585 consecutively treated arches. The International Journal of Prosthodontics. 2018;**31**(5):425-435

[57] Delgado-Ruiz R, Romanos G. Potential causes of titanium particle and ion release in implant dentistry: A systematic review. International Journal of Molecular Sciences. 2018;**13, 19**(11)

[58] Noronha Oliveira M, Schunemann WVH, Mathew MT, Henriques B, Magini RS, Teughels W, et al. Can degradation products released from dental implants affect peri-implant tissues? Journal of Periodontal Research. 2018;**53**:1-11

[59] Wennerberg A, Ide-Ektessabi A, Hatkamata S, Sawase T, Johansson C, Albrektsson T, et al. Titanium release from implants prepared with different surface roughness. An in vitro and in vivo study. Clinical Oral Implants Research. 2004;**15**:505-512

[60] Bressan E, Ferroni L, Gardin C, et al. Metal nanoparticles released from dental implant surfaces: Potential contribution to chronic inflammation and peri-implant bone loss. Materials (Basel). 2019;**12**(12)

[61] Coelho PG, Granato R, Marin C, Teixeira HS, Suzuki M, Valverde GB, et al. The effect of different implant macrogeometries and surface treatment in early biomechanical fixation: An experimental study in dogs. Journal of the Mechanical Behavior of Biomedical Materials. 2011;**4**:1974-1981

[62] Geng JP, Ma QS, Xu W, Tan KB, Liu GR. Finite element analysis of four thread-form configurations in a stepped screw implant. Journal of Oral Rehabilitation. 2004;**31**:233-239

[63] Stein AE, McGlmphy EA, Johnston WM, Larsen PE. Effects of implant design and surface roughness on crestal bone and soft tissue levels in the esthetic zone. The International Journal of Oral & Maxillofacial Implants. 2009;**24**:910-919

[64] Schupbach P, Glauser R. The defense architecture of the human periimplant mucosa: A histological study. The Journal of Prosthetic Dentistry. 2007;**97**:15-25

Chapter 3

Excellency of Hydroxyapatite Composite Scaffolds for Bone Tissue Engineering

Mohammad Shariful Islam, Mohammad Abdulla-Al-Mamun, Alam Khan and Mitsugu Todo

Abstract

The hydroxyapatite [HAp, $Ca_{10}(PO_4)_6(OH)_2$] has a variety of applications in bone fillers and replacements due to its excellent bioactivity and osteoconductivity. It comprises the main inorganic component of hard tissues. Among the various approaches, a composite approach using several components like biopolymer, gelatin, collagen, and chitosan in the functionalization of scaffolds with HAp has the prospective to be an engineered biomaterial for bone tissue engineering. HAp composite scaffolds have been developed to obtain a material with different functionalities such as surface reactivity, bioactivity, mechanical strength, and capability of drug or growth factor delivery. Several techniques and processes for the synthesis and fabrication of biocompatible HAp composite scaffolds suitable for bone regeneration are addressed here. Further, this chapter described the excellences of various HAp composite scaffolds used in *in vitro* and *in vivo* experiments in bone tissue engineering.

Keywords: hydroxyapatite, scaffolds, tissue engineering, bioceramics, composite, stem cell

1. Introduction

Recently, regenerated bone grafts have drawn attention as a promising new bone grafting technology for use in tissue engineering [1]. Bone tissue engineering offers an alternative approach for repairing bone defects caused by trauma, malignancies, and congenital diseases [2]. Scaffolds are one of the key factors for bone tissue engineering. The scaffolds act as substrates by providing a temporary home for growth and proliferation of cells. The scaffolds also provide structural and mechanical support for cell growth. Therefore, scaffolds should possess sufficient mechanical strength to provide structural support and a porous structure to guide new bone tissue in-growth [1, 3, 4]. Hydroxyapatite (HAp) has been used in regenerative science dates back to the 1950s as an inert scaffold for filling of the bone defects [5]. It is a calcium phosphate bioceramic [$Ca_{10}(PO_4)_6(OH)_2$] that has widely been applied as scaffolds in bone tissue engineering because of high osteoconductivity and biocompatibility. It is a well-known bioceramic found as a major component of bone and tooth [6, 7]. HAp is one of the popular bioceramics used in bone tissue engineering because it possesses chemical structure very similar to carbonate apatite which is the major inorganic component of bone [8, 9]. HAp bioceramics have been widely

 IntechOpen

used as artificial bone substitutes because of their favorable biological properties, which include biocompatibility, bioaffinity, bioactivity, and osteoconduction [10]. HAp bioceramics contain only calcium and phosphate ions, and therefore, no adverse local or systemic toxicity has been reported in any study.

In tissue engineering, the interactions between tissue and HAp are important. Therefore, it is necessary to understand the *in vivo* host responses for HAp. Generally, the mechanism of action of a biomaterial is considered to be biocompatible, bioinert, biotolerant, and bioactive and includes bioresorbable materials. Bioactive materials form a chemical bond. The roughness and biomaterial porosity is considered to be an important factor for bonding. In this connection, HAp has displayed an ability to bond directly with the bone. It also exhibits the property of osteoinductivity [10, 11]. HAp scaffolds are very much recognized because of their osteoconduction and osteoinduction properties. Due to the provocation of the host mesenchymal stem cells, osteoinduction takes place in bone graft implantation. Therefore, these stem cells are then distinguished into bone-developing osteoblasts. Wide-ranging researches from worldwide have been accompanied several researches to recognize the osteoinduction potential of HAp over the past numerous years. As a result, through a number of independent studies in several hosts such as dogs, goats, and baboons osteoinduction has been finally detected [11–14]. In relation to the previous development, recently, comprehensive studies have been performed to construct biomimetic scaffolds materials for bone tissue engineering utilizations. Three-dimensional structure of these biomaterials is very much necessary for proper functioning. Few excellent properties of these scaffolds such as a high volume of open and interconnected pores, a bioresorbable scaffold with controlled resorption, appropriate mechanical properties, biocompatibility, and bioactivity are highly recommended in bone tissue engineering [15].

Various permeable scaffolds can be assembled by using both bioactive ceramics and biocompatible polymers for the application in bone tissue engineering [1]. The bioactivity of graft substitutes is mostly governed by the degree of porosity of the fabricated biomaterials, which controls the rate of bone regeneration, local environment, and equilibrium of new bone at the repair site. Therefore, the osteoconductivity of the inductivity potential of the bone graft is synergistically promoted by the pore interconnectivity, geometry, topography, and porosity modulate osteogenesis of the fabricated scaffolds [16–18]. Bioactive ceramics have a chemical composition resembling that of natural bone, allowing osteogenesis and providing bony contact and bonds with host bone [6, 19]. HAp is a typical bioceramic clinically used as a bone substitute, and it has also been used as scaffold materials in bone tissue engineering owing to its bioactivity, biocompatibility, and osteoconductivity. However, the low strength and toughness of HAp has limited its wide application in orthopedic implants [20]. The main reason for these low mechanical properties is thought to be the decomposition of HAp into different calcium phosphate phases, such as tricalcium phosphate (TCP) and even tetracalcium phosphate (TTCP) [21]. Therefore, the mechanical properties of the HAp porous scaffold must be enhanced to use effectively in load-bearing compartments and tissue engineering applications. Various kinds of natural polymers, synthetic polymers (chitosan), protein (collagen), and bioceramics have been used along with HAp to develop composite porous scaffolds for bone tissue engineering in recent years.

2. Synthesis and fabrication processes

Scaffold fabricated by various methods acts as a substrate to stimulate cell adhesion, maintenance of differentiated cell function without hampering proliferation. It is also a template to establish and direct the growth of cells and help in the construction of extracellular matrix (ECM) [22]. Therefore, a biodegradable scaffold serves as a temporary skeleton in bone tissue engineering. Generally, when such scaffolds are inserted into the sites of faulty or lost bone to support and stimulate bone tissue regeneration, they gradually degrades and is replaced by new bone tissue [23–25]. The use of HAp as a scaffold material has been introduced in bone tissue engineering mainly due to its unique properties and similarity with bone components. The low strength and toughness of HAp has limited its wide application in bone tissue engineering. Therefore, improved mechanical properties of the HAp porous scaffolds are required for the extensive range of applications and effective utilization in load-bearing compartments [1]. To overcome the brittleness of HAp porous body, biodegradable synthetic polymers such as poly (lactic co-glycolic acid) (PLGA), para-Methoxy-N-methylamphetamine (PMMA), poly(L-lactic acid) PLLA, and poly(ε-caprolactone) PCL are used as composites [26–29]. Even some attempts have been made to introduce bioceramics into polymer-based scaffolds or to combine synthetic polymers with natural polymers to enhance their biological capacity [30]. Recently, several studies are focusing on the development of HAp-COL and HAp-COL/HAp composite scaffolds or HA-CNT nanocomposites with improved mechanical properties [31, 32]. HAp-COL and HAp-COL/HAp composite scaffolds or HA-CNT nanocomposites for orthopedic implants are synthesizing through template method, plasma spraying, laser surface alloying, electrophoretic deposition, and aerosol deposition [31, 33–37]. In addition to conventional sintering and hot isostatic pressing, spark plasma sintering (SPS) has also been employed to fabricate freestanding HA-CNT composites [38–41]. HAp-COL and HAp-COL/HAp composite scaffolds are also fabricated in a specific freeze-drying procedure [31].

2.1 Synthesis of HAp porous scaffolds by the template method

A template method (using polyurethane foam [PU]) was applied to prepare HAp porous scaffolds from HAp slurry. The HAp slurry was synthesized from HAp nanopowder and a 5 wt% solution of polyvinyl alcohol (PVA) (Wako Pure Chemical Industries, Ltd.). The HAp slurry was prepared by mixing the HAp powder and PVA solution at a mixing ratio of 1:1 (1 g of HAp to 1 ml of PVA) using a centrifuge mixing machine (Imoto Co, Ltd.). The machine was kneading for 10 minutes and degassing (removal of gas bubbles) for 8 minutes to obtain the best outcome. A PU sponge sheet (HR-30, Bridgestone) was cut into cubic templates with dimensions of 10 × 10 × 10 mm. These cubes were then immersed into the ready HAp slurry. To escape blockage of the pores by the slurry, the additional slurry was removed by pressing the cubes at compression ratios of 50, 75, and 95%. To eliminate water content and to attach the HAp powders to the surface of the sponge framework, the cubes were then dried out at room temperature for 24 hours. The dried cubes were then calcined at 400°C for 6 hours and further sintered at 1000, 1100, or 1200°C for 3 hours. The heating rate was set to 10°C/minute. The solidified samples were termed "pure HAp scaffolds" thereafter. The sintering process is illustrated schematically in **Figure 1(a)** [1].

2.2 Fabrication of HAp porous scaffolds with collagen and HAp particles

In a collagen-1 solution prepared, pure HAp scaffolds were dipped (Nippon Meat Packers Inc., Osaka, Japan) and then it was vacuumed for at least 30 minutes to eliminate the excess air. To synthesize HAp scaffolds with collagen coating, firstly, the surplus collagen solution was removed manually by pipette, and then the samples were dried at room temperature for at least 48 hours. On the other hand, a milk-like slime of HAp particles was formulated by mixing it accurately with the collagen-1 solution

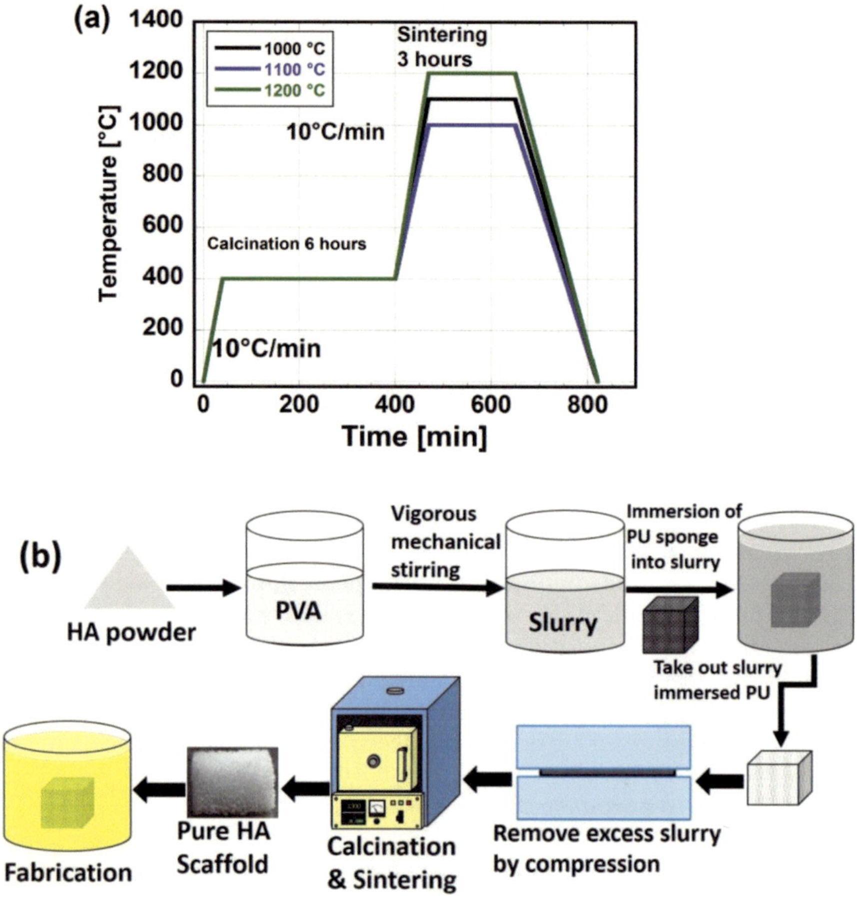

Figure 1.
Schematic of the (a) sintering processes and (b) synthesis to the fabrication of HAp porous composite scaffolds [1].

(1:9) at 30°C and stirred continuously by a magnetic stirrer. To fabricate HAp scaffolds with collagen-HAp coating, the prepared slime was then poured over the pure HAp scaffolds. After that, the additional slime was removed and the scaffolds were dried out for at least 48 hours to get fabricate HAp scaffolds. The two distinct types of fabricated composite scaffolds were thereafter termed as "HAp-COL" and "HAp-COL/HAp particle-coated scaffolds," respectively. The detail fabrication processes of the HAp-COL and HAp-COL/HAp scaffolds are illustrated schematically here in **Figure 1(b)** [1]. Further, a specific freeze-drying procedure was applied to fabricate coated HAp scaffolds form both types. The pure HAp porous composite scaffolds were frozen at −20°C for 24 hours and then freeze-dried at −50°C for 24 hours. These samples were termed "HAp-Collagen or HAp-Collagen/HAp particles two-phase scaffolds" [31].

2.3 Fabrication of HAp composite by Nd-YAG laser

HAp composite scaffolds were fabricated by a unique process where HAp powders were coated on titanium substrates at low temperature, and this coating/substrate interfacing was enhanced by a laser surface engineering. In this technology, Nd-YAG laser was transmitted to HAp powders and the laser power was absorbed by titanium substrate to produce a thin layer of the molten region. Finally, in this procedure, HAp powders were kept at low temperature before they were entrapped in the metallic layer during coating [35].

2.4 Fabrication of HAp composite by electrophoretic deposition (EPD)

Usually, various bioactive ceramics like HAp are coated containing carbon nanotubes on metallic substrates through electrophoretic deposition. The EPD technique is described by Sing et al.. Using EPD, a variety of potentially bioactive ceramic coatings constructed on combinations of either HAp or titanium oxide nanoparticles with carbon nanotubes (CNTs) have been deposited on metallic substrates. Further, sol-gel-derived ultrafine HAp powders (10–70 nm) were dispersed in multi-wall nanotube-containing ethanol suspensions maintained at pH = ~3.5 and successfully coated onto Ti alloy wires at 20 V for 1–3 minutes. Commercially available TiO2 nanopowders and surface-treated CNTs in aqueous suspensions were co-deposited on stainless steel planar substrates for TiO2/CNT coatings. A field strength of 20 V/cm and a deposition time of 4 minutes were used in this process to work at pH = 5 [36].

2.5 Fabrication of HAp composite by aerosol deposition

Hahn et al. developed an aerosol deposition technique to fabricate HAp-carbon nanotube (CNT) composite coatings on Ti plate. Through this aerosol deposition technique, authors fabricating HAp-CNT powders composites for biomedical applications. For the deposition process, HAp-CNT powder mixtures with CNT contents of 1 and 3 wt.% were used. Dense coatings with a thickness of 5 μm were fabricated, irrespective of the content of CNTs. The propagation and alkaline phosphatase (ALP) activity of MC3T3-E1 pre-osteoblast cells grown on the HAp-CNT composite coatings was estimated. A higher propagation and alkaline phosphatase (ALP) activity of MC3T3-E1 pre-osteoblast cells grown on the fabricated HAp-CNT composite coatings was detected than those on the bare Ti and pure HAp coating. It was also found that by increasing the CNT content of the composite materials, an enhanced ALP activity of the composite coatings was obtained. Therefore, the findings suggested that for the improvement both the mechanical and biological performances of HAp coatings, CNTs would be an effective fortifying agent [37].

2.6 Fabrication of HAp composite by in situ chemical vapor deposition

Li et al. described a novel process to fabricate carbon nanotubes (CNTs) (Fe)/HAp composite. By this novel process (CNTs), (Fe)/HAp composite was successfully prepared where CNTs homogeneously dispersed. In this procedure, at first Fe_2O_3/HAp precursor was produced and then calcined in an atmosphere of N_2 gas. The reduction reaction was done in the presence of hydrogen of the Fe_2O_3/HAp precursor to yield Fe/HAp catalyst, and finally, in situ synthesis of nanotubes by chemical vapor deposition over Fe/HAp catalyst was performed. To yield CNTs (Fe)/HAp bulk composites, these outstanding CNTs (Fe)/HAp composite powder was utilized. These CNTs (Fe)/HAp bulk composites further pressed and sintered to produce CNTs (Fe)/HAp nanocomposites. It was analyzed that the CNTs distributed homogenously and bonded strongly with the HAp matrix [39].

2.7 Fabrication of HAp composite by poly(ε-caprolactone) (PCL) and poly(L-lactide) (PLLA)

PCL pallets with the molecular formula $(CH2)_5CO_2$, molecular weight (Mw) of 10^5g.mol^{-1}, glass transition temperature Tg = −62.62°C, and melting point Tm = 65.4°C (Celgreen PH7, Daicel Chemistry Industries Co., Ltd.) were dissolved

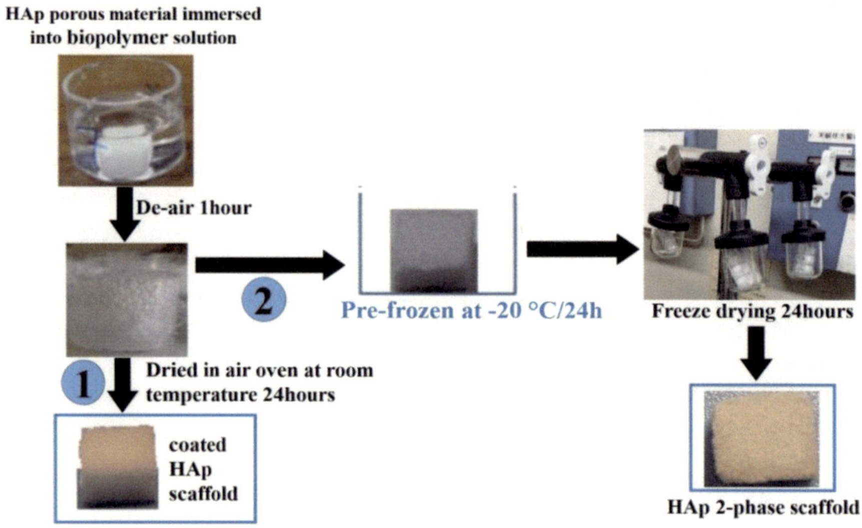

Figure 2.
Schematic of biopolymer-reinforced HAp porous materials.

in 1,4 dioxane (Kishida Chemical Co., Ltd., Osaka, Japan) to get the solution with a concentration of 1, 3, 5, 7 and 10 wt% by stirring at 60°C for 2 hours. HAp porous scaffolds were dipped into the solution, and it was then vacuumed for 1 hour to eliminate the air. For drying of these scaffolds, two different conditions were applied. The drenched HAp porous scaffolds were taken out from the PCL solution and then dried in an air oven at room temperature for 24 hours in the first drying process. These specimens were named as "HAp/PCL-coated scaffolds." On the other hand, in the second drying process, the freeze-drying procedure was employed to obtain a two-phase porous construction. After excess PCL solution was removed from the soaked HAp porous materials, the samples were frozen at −20°C for 24 hours and then freeze-dried at −50°C for 24 hours. These specimens were named as "HAp/PCL 2-phase scaffolds." The summary of the reinforcement process is shown in **Figure 2** [42].

3. Excellences in bone tissue engineering

The scaffolds act as a temporary substitute in bone tissue engineering and the interest of researchers in it as it permits mechanical support until the tissue has regenerated and remodeled itself naturally. It is well established that biopolymers such as collagen [43], chitosan [44], and hyaluronic acid [45]; biodegradable synthetic polymers such as poly(L-lactic acid) [46], poly(ε-caprolactone) [47], and polyglycolic acid (PGA) [48]; and bioactive ceramics such as hydroxyapatite [49], α-tricalcium phosphates [50], and β-tricalcium phosphates (β-TCP) [51] are used as the raw materials for the preparation of the scaffolds suitable for tissue engineering. These materials have been independently used to develop scaffolds, but composite materials have also been considered as ideal materials having mechanical stability, biocompatibility, cell proliferation, and easy proccessability [52–55]. However, HAp grows interested in scientists and researchers due to its mechanical and biological response and its efficiency in repairing a hard tissue defect in the composite state. This section will summarize the excellence of different HAp composite scaffolds for bone substitutes and hard tissue repair.

3.1 *In vitro* experiments using HAp composite scaffolds

Phanny (in our lab) conducted a study using HAp/PCL-coated scaffold and HAp/PCL two-phase scaffold to investigate the mechanical properties variation, biocompatibility, and differentiation efficiency within 4 weeks of cell culture in a standard medium and osteoblast differentiation medium [42]. Human mesenchymal stem cells (hMSCs) were seeded in both types of scaffold for 1–4 weeks with an α-minimum essential medium eagle with L-glutamine and phenol red (MEMα) for the growth and with osteoblast differentiation medium for cellular differentiation. The author reported that both HAp/PCL-coated scaffold (**Figure 3**, left) and HAp/PCL two-phase scaffolds were biocompatible where hMSCs have grown and proliferated rapidly (**Figure 3**, right). The level of p-nitrophenol obtained via ALP assay of both types of scaffolds are almost the same because the cells tended to proliferate in standard medium rather than differentiation. The cells cultured in osteoblast differentiation medium were able to differentiate into an osteoblastic lineage with an increasing level of p-nitrophenol and density of ARS staining. It was also found that specimens without cell seeding continuously decreased in both elastic modulus and compressive strength in both standard medium and osteoblast differentiation medium and remained lower than that of specimens with cell culture.

Therefore, it was concluded that the ability to allow cells to grow, proliferate, differentiate, and maintain mechanical properties of HAp/PCL-coated and two-phase scaffolds are a high potential candidate for bone tissue engineering applications [42].

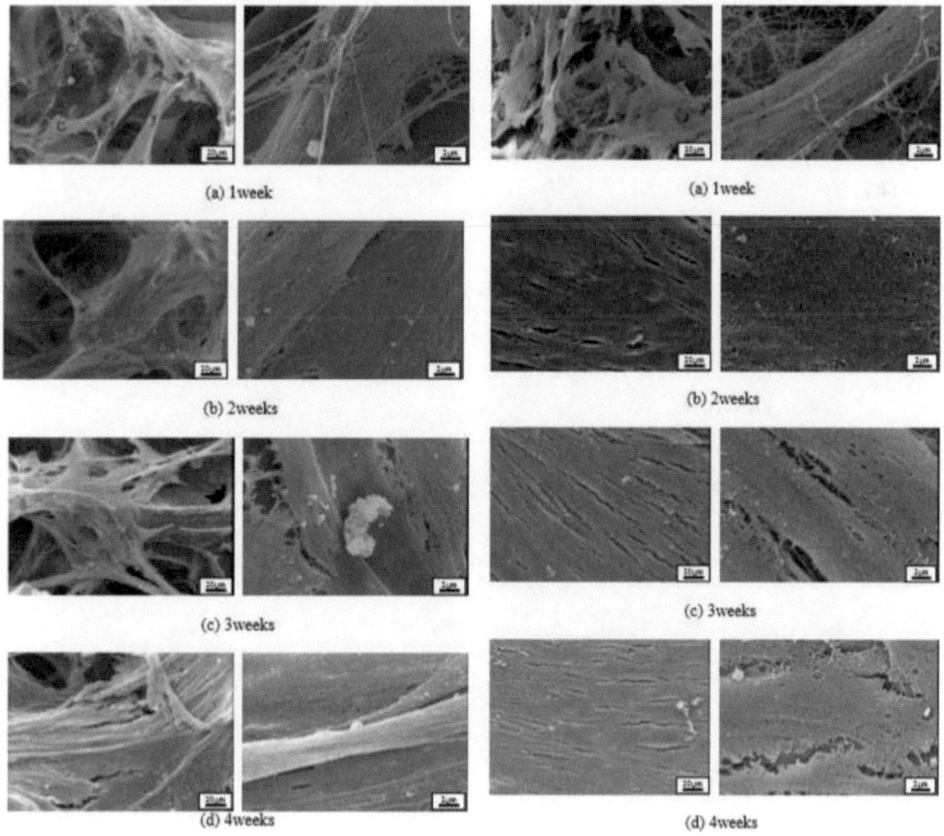

Figure 3.
FE-SEM images of the morphology of cell growth on HAp/PCL-coated (left) and HAp/PCL two-phase scaffolds (right).

It was reported in our previous study that hMSCs could be successfully cultured over HAp-COL and HAp-COL/HAp scaffolds. It was confirmed from that evaluation that the scaffolds exhibited the best performance in terms of mechanical properties at a 50% compressive ratio. **Figure 4** represents the FE-SEM micrographs of the surface regions of composite scaffolds with hMSCs [1]. In this figure, hMSCs's adhesion and proliferation behaviors up to 7 days of culturing were observed on the surfaces. The FE-SEM micrographs of hMSCs cultivated over the fabricated composite scaffolds of HAp-COL and HAp-COL/HAp sintered at 1000, 1100, and 1200°C are shown in figures (a), (c), and (e), and (b), (d), and (f), respectively. Most cells adhered tightly to the surface and were well disseminated. These results indicated that the composite scaffolds had favorable bioactivity for the promotion of cell adhesion and proliferation far excelling than that of pure HAp scaffolds. The effects of the compressive ratio and sintering temperature on cell-scaffold interactions were evaluated through a cell proliferation assay using a cell-counting kit up to 14 days of culture.

The growth performance of hMSCs over the constructed porous composite scaffolds is exhibited in **Figure 5**. Primarily, 1×10^4 cells were seeded on the fabricated porous composite scaffolds. After the cells seeding well, the cell proliferation

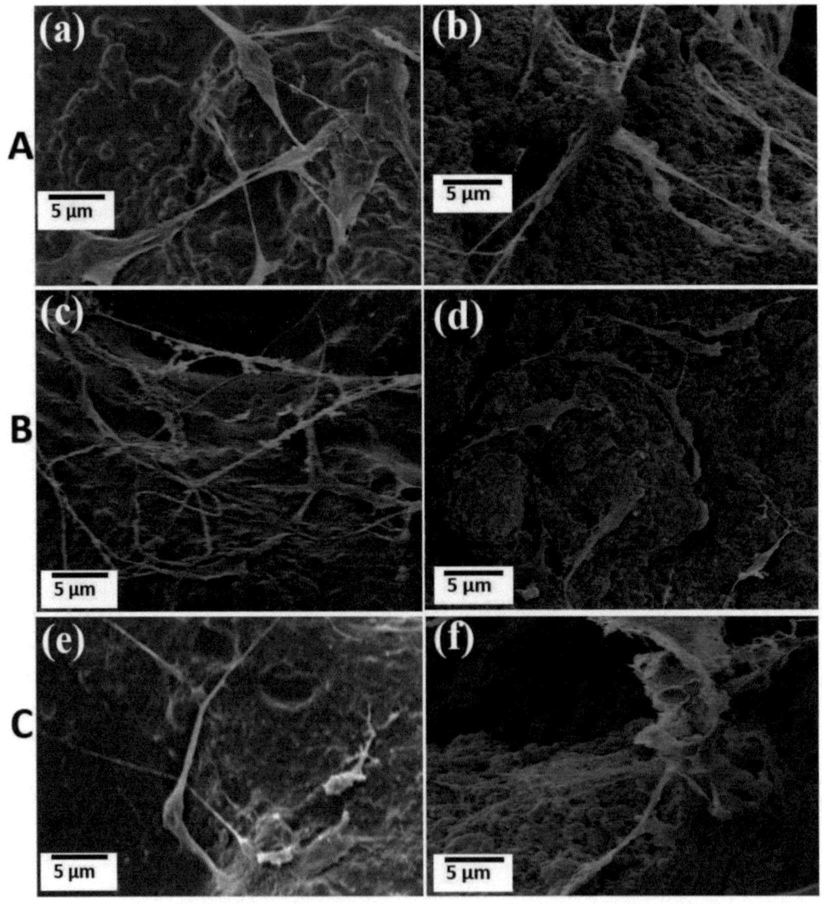

Figure 4.
The FE-SEM images of 7 days culture period of hMSCs over HAp-COL and HAp-COL/HAp porous composite scaffolds fabricated at a 50% compressive ratio and sintered at (A) 1000C, (B) 1100°C, and (C) 1200°C. the FE-SEM images HAp-COL and HAp-COL/HAp porous composite scaffolds are represented by (a), (c), and (e) and (b), (d), and (f) at sintering temperature 1000°C, 1100°C, and 1200°C, respectively [1].

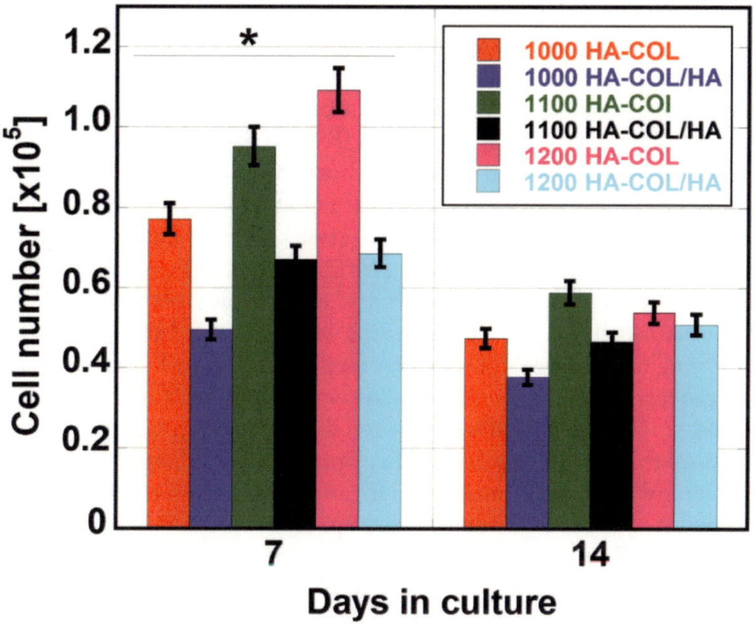

Figure 5.
The proliferation of hMSCs in HAp-COL and HAp-COL/HAp composite scaffolds fabricated at a 50% compressive ratio and sintered at 1000, 1100, and 1200°C with up to 14 days of culture. Each set of data represents the mean ± SD, n = 6, $^{*}p < 0.05$ *[1].*

behavior was recorded at 7 and 14 days of culture. It was noteworthy that the cell number increased until 7 days of culture for all types of scaffolds, while cell multiplication declined as the culturing days continued. The growth performance of hMSCs over the HAp-COL scaffolds sintered at 1000, 1100, and 1200°C displayed distinctive trend over their counterparts [1].

Wahl and Czernuszka summarized and compared a few excellent reports of *in vitro* experiments using HAp composite scaffolds and are listed here in **Table 1** [56].

3.2 *In vivo* experiments using HAp composite scaffolds

Cai et al. fabricated coral hydroxyapatite (CHAp) as a cuboid of 5 mm × 5 mm × 10 mm with an inclined groove. In this study, the prepared CHAp biomaterials was highly porous (porosity: 30–70%) with a fully interconnected pore with an average pore diameter of 100–600 μm. Here, the induced BMSCs

Composites	Cell culturing or implantation	Period (new tissue formed)
HA-Collagen (Du et al.) [57]	Bone extract wrapped around composite osteogenic cells	21 days (mineralized bone)
HA-Collagen (Clarke et al.) [58]	Human-derived bone cell culture	32 days (connective tissue and mineralized bone)
HA-Collagen (Wu et al.) [59]	Osteoblasts from rat calvaria	21 days (mineralized bone)
HA-Collagen (Wang et al.) [60]	Chondrocytes in a closed chamber	49 days (cartilage)
HA-Collagen-Elastin (Rovira et al.) [61]	Osteoblasts from trabecular bone	15 days (mineralized bone)

Table 1.
In vitro *experiments in bone tissue engineering using different HAp composites.*

were seeded on sterilized CHAp scaffold by a concentration of 20 × 10^6 cells/ml (200 ± 17 μL/scaffold, about 4 × 10^6 cells/scaffold) and were 3D cultured for 1 week before implantation. The growth behavior of BMSCs on the CHAp scaffold was assessed by using a scanning electron microscope and confocal laser electronic microscope [62]. The authors described an effective methodology to generate bone tissue and healing bone defect in ectopic and orthotopic sites. In this methodology, a tissue-engineered bone flap with a vascular pedicle of saphenous arteriovenous with an organized vascular network was observed after 4 weeks of implantation and followed by a successful repair of the fibular defect in beagle dogs (**Figure 6**).

Engineered bone formation in ectopic and orthotopic sites after implantation of 9 months over four CHAp scaffold groups were evaluated by CT (computed tomography) analysis. The stimuluses of vascularization and micro-environment on tissue-engineered bone were quantitatively analyzed by the comparison of bone formation and scaffold degradation between different groups (**Figure 7**). The results indicated that in the first 3 months, vascularization improved engineered bone formation by 2 times of non-vascular group and bone defect micro-environment improved it by 3 times the ectopic group, and the CHAp scaffold degradation was enhanced as well [62]. In the VSC group, the HE staining of decalcified paraffin sections after 3 months embedding exhibited that there was a minor volume of bone-like tissue developed at the surface of the CHAp scaffold (**Figure 7(B)**). **Figure 7(C)** and **(D)** indicates the gradual improvement of engineered bone tissue after 6 months and a well-developed Haversian system with little residual scaffold remaining after 9 months, respectively. In the SC group, after 3 months of implantation, only the osteoid was shown and until 6 months of implantation, there was no significant bone formation, but after 9 months of implantation, engineered bone tissue enlarged with much residual scaffold (**Figure 7(E)–(H)**). **Figure 7(I)–(P)** denotes the gradual degradation of the CHAp scaffolds without bone formation in both VS and S groups, the pores of the majority of CHAp scaffold fill with fibrous connective tissue and a large number of inflammatory cells. Moreover, more typical vascular structures and less inflammatory cells were seen in the VS group than that in the S group (**Figure 7L** and **P**).

In another study, Kikuchi et al. (2001) fabricated a biodegradable hydroxyapatite/collagen (HAp/Col) nanocomposite [63]. In this method, through the lyophilization of the precipitate of HAp/Col composites, HAp/Col powder was formulated. About 0.5 g of the prepared HAp/Col powder was well mixed with 3 ml of 0.9% NaCl solution (Wako, Japan) and 35 Al of 5 M CaCO3 (Wako). In a 0.9% NaCl

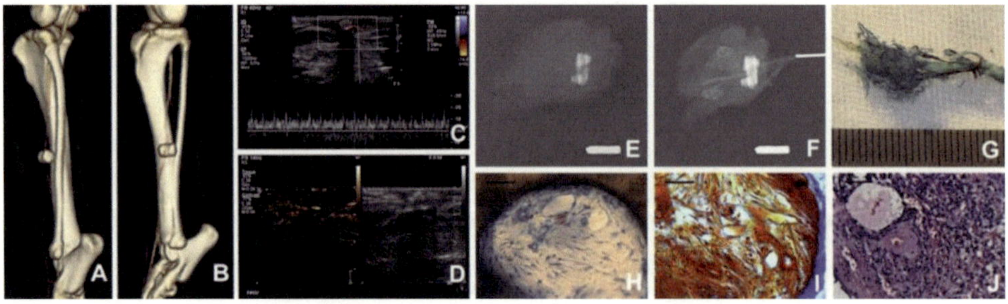

Figure 6.
Representation of the vascularization over MSC coral hydroxyapatite scaffold using cell-CHA constructs at 4 weeks post-implantation. Here, (A) and (B) represent CT angiography and (C) and (D) indicate ultrasonic inspection. Further, (E) and (F) indicate X-ray before and after vascular corrosion cast and (G) represent vascular corrosion cast. HE and Masson's trichrome staining of cell-CHA constructs in undecalcification sections and decalcification sections is indicated by (H), (I), and (J), respectively. Scale bars: 10 mm (F), (G), 50 mm (H)–(J) [62].

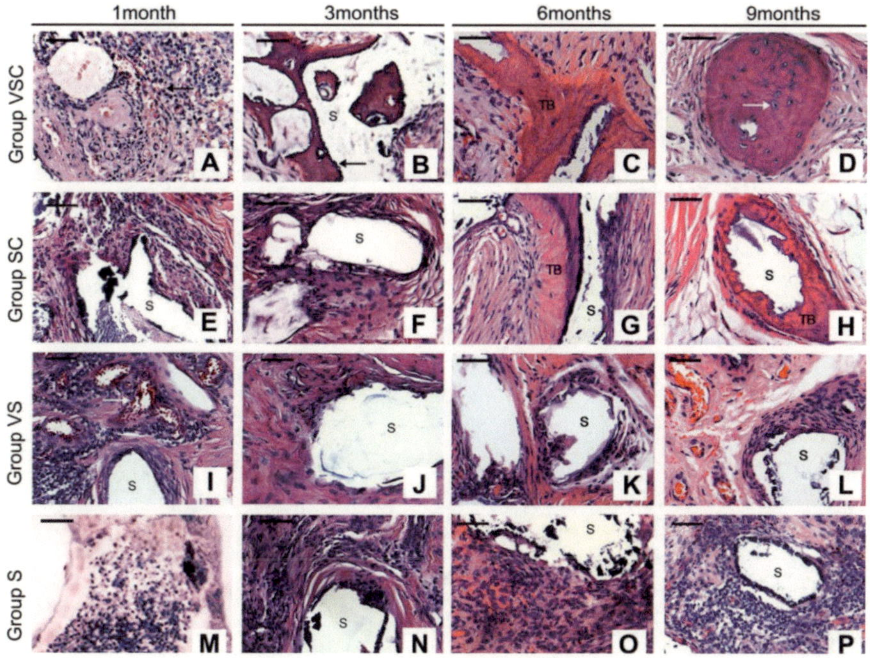

Figure 7.
Histological observation of different CHAp-scaffold constructs implanted into spatium intramuscular of the hind limb at 1, 3, 6, and 9 months post-implantation (HE staining; S, CHA scaffold; TB, tissue-engineered bone). Scale bars: 50 mm. Here, HE staining of decalcified paraffin sections is showed. In VSC group, bone-like tissue formation at the surface of the CHA scaffold after 1 and 3 months implantation are indicated by plate (A) and (B), respectively; gradual increase of engineered bone tissue after 6 months and visible well-developed Haversian system after 9 months implantation are indicated by plate (C) and (D), respectively. In SC group, visible osteoid after 3 months, no significant bone formation until 6 months and engineered bone tissue increased with much residual scaffold remaining after 9 months implantation are represented by (E), (F), (G), and (H), respectively. Filling the pores of the CHA scaffolds in both VS and S groups with fibrous connective tissue and a large number of inflammatory cells indicated by (I–P).

solution, 1.5 ml of 3% sodium alginate (Wako) was added, dissolved, and mixed. D-gluconic acid lactone (60 mg, Sigma, USA) was added to the HAp/Col-alginate mixture to initiate gelation, and the mixture was injected into a mold and left for 45 minutes at room temperature. The composite has a bone-like nanostructure; the length of the HAp crystals is up to 50 nm. The authors investigated the capability of HAp/Col-alginate as a bone filler in the rat femur and as a carrier of BMP using an ectopic bone formation model (**Figure 8**). Vigorous bone growth around the fabricated scaffolds and tissue invasion into these scaffolds was observed during the experiment. A comparison was made between those observed for simple alginate and porous HAp. Furthermore, HAp/Col-alginate was investigated as a carrier of recombinant human bone morphogenetic protein 2 (rh-BMP2). It was revealed that bone formation throughout the implant 5 weeks after implantation without obvious deformation of the material was obtained by using the HAp/Col-alginate (20 μl) with the rh-BMP2 (100 μg/ml, 15 μl), whereas bone development was detected only in a part of a squashed collagen sponge [64]. In **Figure 8 (A–C)**, prominent bone formation of the HAp/Col-alginate treated with the 100 μg/ml BMP solution was remarkably extended throughout almost the whole implant, and bone marrow-like tissue also developed. It was noticed that the implants shrank when there was no bone formation. Further, it was observed that ectopic bone formation was obtained using collagen sponge treated with the 100 μg/ml of rh-BMP2 solution, but new bone had not extended all through the implant even after 5 weeks (**Figure 8(D)**) [64].

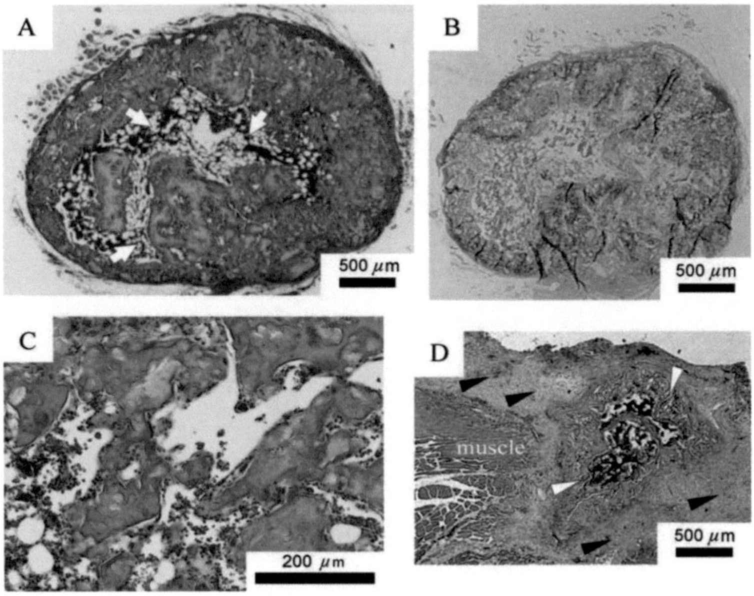

Figure 8.
BMP2 (100 μg/ml) induced ectopic bone formation after 5 weeks of implantation. Here, (A–C) denote HAp/col-alginate with BMP; (A), (B), (C), and (D) stand for HE section of the whole implant, immunostaining section with antiosteocalcin, higher magnification, and collagen sponge with BMP, respectively. Here, bone marrow-like tissue was indicated by white arrows. Further, black arrowheads and white arrowheads indicate soft and bone, respectively [64].

Ripamonti et al. conducted spontaneous induction research of bone formation in heterotopic *rectus abdominis* and orthotopic calvarial sites by coral-derived biomimetic matrices of different chemical compositions. The authors conducted a long-term study in the non-human primate *Papio ursinus*. In this methodology, rods (diameter 20 mm × and 7 mm) were implanted in heterotopic *rectus abdominis* sites; discs (diameter 25 mm) were implanted in orthotopic calvarial defects of six adult non-human primates, *P. ursinus.* Fully converted hydroxyapatite replicas sintered at 1100°C were used as heterotopic samples. These fully converted hydroxyapatite replicas were coated with the synthetic peptide P15 known to increase the adhesion of fibroblasts to an organic bovine mineral to further enhance the spontaneous osteoinductive activity. Thereafter, bone induction was evaluated by a histological examination, alkaline phosphatase, and osteocalcin expression, as well as by the expression of BMP-7, GDF-10, and collagen type IV mRNAs at 60, 90, and 365 days. Bone induction occurred in the concavities of the scaffolds matrices at all time points. It was evident of bone marrow formation in the P15-coated and uncoated implants at 365 days. Moreover, resorption of partially converted calcium carbonate/hydroxyapatite and remodeling of the newly formed bone was apparent. The northern blot analyses of samples from heterotopic specimens indicated high levels of expression of BMP-7 and collagen type IV mRNA in all samples at 60 days. Therefore, it was correlating with the induction of the osteoblastic phenotype in invading fibrovascular cells. Expanded bone formation across the different implanted constructs of the orthotopic samples was also observed (**Figure 9**).

The concavities of the biomimetic matrices and the remodeling cycle of the osteogenic primate cortico-cancellous bone stimulate the ripple-like cascade of the induction of bone formation. It is demonstrated for the first time through this study that spontaneous differentiation of bone was induced by partially converted HAp/CC constructs. It was noted that this bone induction was only seen 1 year post-implantation [12].

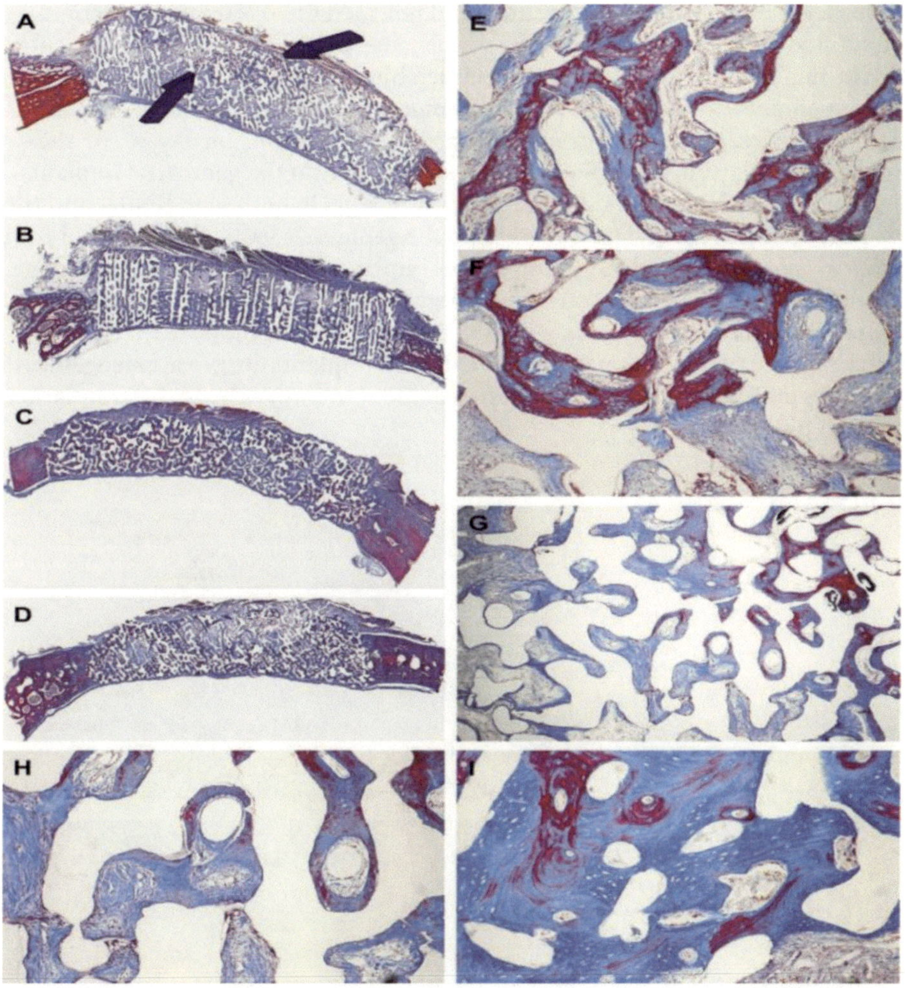

Figure 9.
Demonstration of calvarial incorporation of 13% hydroxyapatite/calcium carbonate paradigms collected on 60 (A, E, F), 90 (B, F, G, H), and 365 days (C, D, and I) after implantation in calvarial defects of Papio ursinus. *Here, (a) stands for islands of newly formed bone (blue arrows) scattered within the internal and central regions of the implanted coral-derived construct; (E and F) stand for the induction of bone formation within the porous spaces of the implanted biomimetic matrices; (B, F, G, and H) stand for induction of bone formation in porous biomimetic constructs harvested 90 days after implantation in calvarial defects. Further, (C, D, and I) denote calvarial constructs harvested on day 365 after implantation showing significant induction of bone formation with solid blocks (I) of newly formed bone [12].*

Ripamonti et al. also fabricated osteoinductive titanium implants for the induction of bone formation. The experimental titanium implants were prepared with a sequence of 36 repetitive concavities. The estimated diameter, depth, and space distance of these concavities was 1600, 800, and 1000 μm, respectively. To prepare edentulous mandibular ridges for later implantation, mandibular molars and premolars were taken out. After a healing period of 7–8 months, in the left and right, edentulized hemi-mandibles planar and geometric hydroxyapatite-coated titanium constructs were entrenched, respectively. In this study, three planar and three geometric implants were implanted in the left and right tibiae, respectively; additionally, planar and geometric constructs were also inserted in the *rectus abdominis* muscle. A total of six animals were euthanized at 30 and 90 days after implantation for this study; one animal was euthanized 5 days after surgery, and the remaining animal was euthanized 31 months after implantation. Undecalcified longitudinal sections were precision-sawed, ground, and polished to 40–60 μm; all sections were stained with a modified Goldner's trichrome. By the EXAKT precision cutting and grinding system, undecalcified specimen block preparation was accomplished. Histomorphometric analyses of bone in contact (BIC) revealed that there was no difference between the geometric *vs*. planar control implants on day 30; on the other hand, on day 90, the ratio of BIC to surface within the geometric implants was greater than that of the standard planar implants in both mandibular and tibial sites. Further, selected concavities cut into the geometric implants harvested from the *rectus abdominis* muscle 31 months after implantation exhibited the spontaneous induction of bone formation with mineralized bone surfaced by osteoid seams (**Figure 10**). Therefore, these data in non-human primates indicate that geometrically constructed plasma-sprayed titanium implants are *per se* osteogenic, the concavities providing a unique microenvironment to initiate bone differentiation by induction [65].

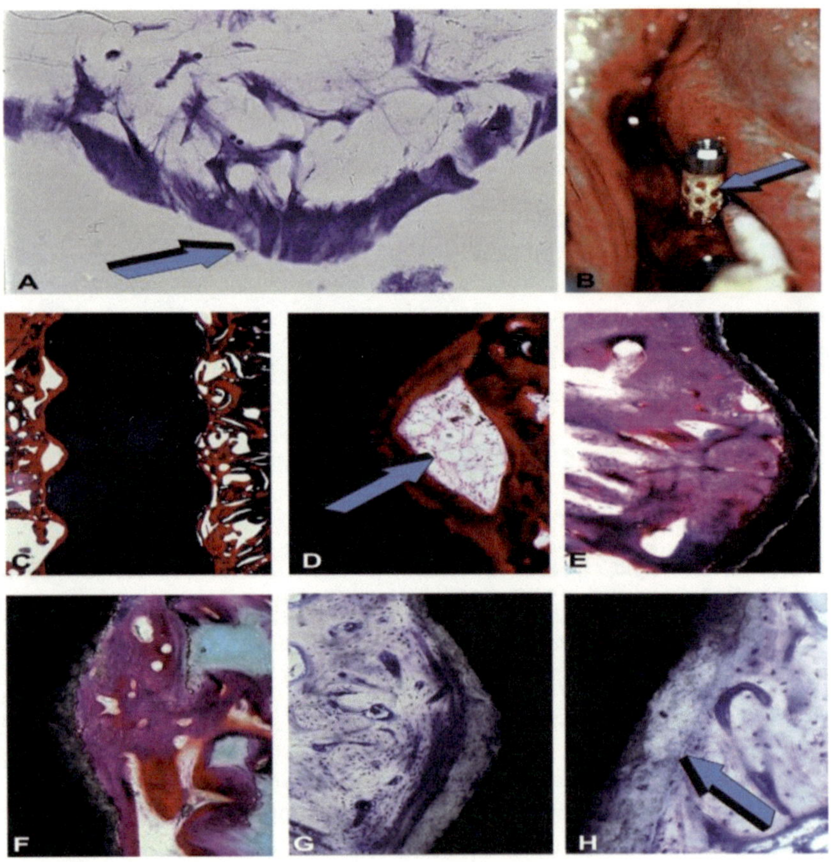

Figure 10.
Tissue evolution, induction, remodeling, and osteointegration within the in vivo *bioreactor of the concavities 90 days after implantation within the edentulized hemi-mandibles of the non-human primate* Papio ursinus. *Here, (A) denotes the instrumental for the preparation of the geometric implants, attachment, orientation, and alignment of MC 3 T3-E1 cells* in vitro *within the geometric cue of the concavity of the coral-derived calcium phosphate macroporous construct. (B) Indicates insertion into the edentulous ridge of the non-human primate* P. ursinus, *the concavities of the* in vivo *bioreactor adsorb plasma and plasma products during the surgical procedure (blue arrow) but not the planar linear inter-concavity spaces. Further, osteointegration along the geometric implant with marrow spaces within the concavity osteointegrated space is denoted by (C) and (D) (blue arrow), whereas mineralized remodeled bone tightly integrated with the hydroxyapatite coating, remodeling, and blending into the highly crystalline hydroxyapatite layer are denoted by E, F, G, H, respectively (H blue arrow) [65].*

In a previous study, porous composite biomaterial of hydroxyapatite (HAp) and periosteal graft was used to repair an induced maxillary bone defect where a defect was created in the premaxillary bone of rats. In this study, four groups were used: (1) those treated with the mucoperiosteal graft from the premaxilla, (2) those treated with HAp combined with a mucoperiosteal graft from the premaxilla, (3) those treated with HAp combined with a periosteal graft from the femur, and (4) those treated with a periosteal graft from the femur. It was revealed from the radiographic evaluation from all groups that no signs of bone formation after 2 weeks were detected but radiolucency was found inside the HAp implants after 16 weeks. It was clear that cell proliferation occurred from the periosteum covering the defect. Moreover, bone tissue formation was detected from the defect margin to inside the defect in all cases. Interestingly, after 8 and 16 weeks of implantation, mature bone was observed around the HAp implants (**Figure 11**). Therefore, it was concluded that the periosteal graft provides reasonable support to the HAp implant, allowing the development of new bone [66].

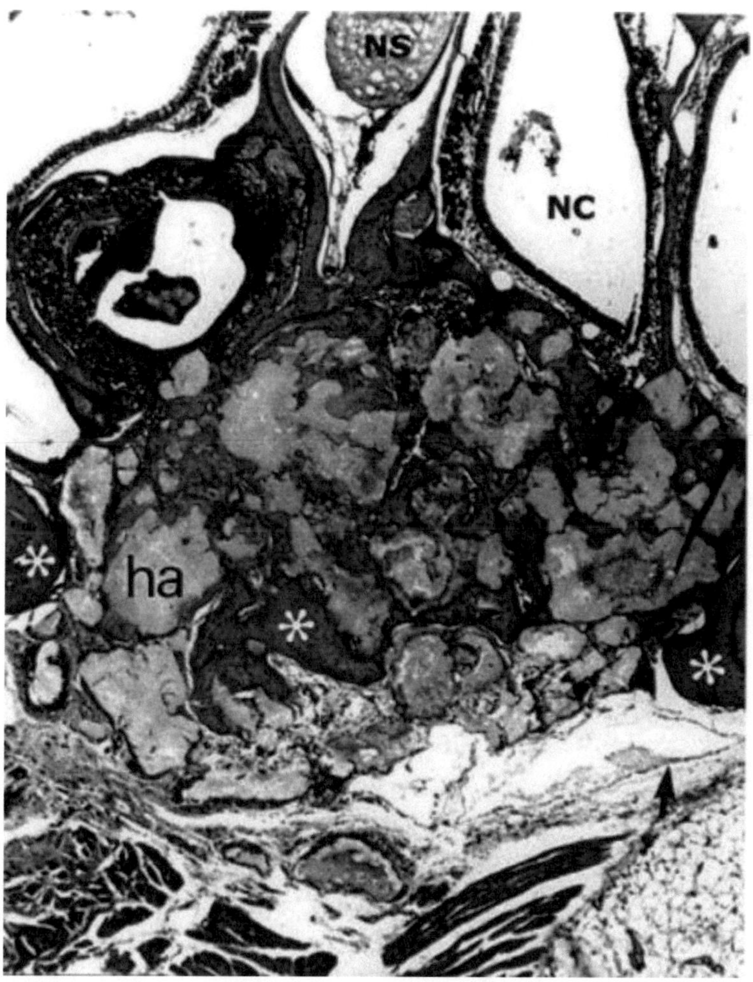

Figure 11.
A histologic frontal section through bone defect covered with mucoperiosteum from the premaxilla combined with HA (group 2). After 16 weeks, the defect in the premaxilla was partially occupied by newly formed bone (white stars) with a mature appearance and by the HA blocks, while there were spaces filled by connective tissue. The mucoperiosteum from the premaxilla remained the HA blocks in the defect (black arrow). (Original magnification 32; hematoxylin-eosin stain).

Composites	Cell culturing or implantation	Period (new tissue formed)
CO3Appatite-Collagen (Okazaki et al.) [67]	Implantation in rat periosteum cranii	21 days (mineralized bone)
PCCA-TCP-Collagen (Du et al.) [68]	Implantation in rat thigh muscle	7 days (connective tissue and capillary vessels)
HA-Collagen (Kikuchi et al.) [69]	Implantation in beagle tibia	54 days (mineralized bone)
HA-Collagen (Itoh et al.) [70]	Implantation in beagle cervical spine	14 days (start of callus formation)
FGMgCO3Ap-Collagen (Yamasaki et al.) [71]	Implantation in rat periosteum cranii	14–28 days (mineralized bone)
HA-Collagen Alginate (Sotome et al.) [64]	Implantation in the rat femur	14 days (mineralized bone)
nHA-Anionic Collagen (Martins and Goissis) [72]	Implantation in rat infraorbital bone	60 days (mineralized bone)
cAP-Collagen (Suh et al.) [73]	Implantation in rabbit skin	98 days (mineralized bone)

Table 2.
In vivo *experiments in bone tissue engineering using different HAp composites.*

Moreover, Wahl and Czernuszka (2006) summarized and compared a few excellent reports of *in vivo* experiments using HAp composite scaffolds and are listed here in **Table 2** [56].

The biodegradable porous scaffolds of HAp synthesized and fabricated by the mentioned methods showed several advantages and disadvantages. The porosity of the HAp scaffolds plays an important role in tissue engineering to control cell functions and to guide the formation of new tissues and organs. Therefore, no matter what the materials are, scaffolds must have sufficient porosity to allow for cellular infiltration and proper cell function [31]. The fabricated pore structures of HAp scaffolds facilitated cell seeding, cell penetration, and distribution in the scaffolds. On the other hand, the bottleneck of the mentioned methods was time-consuming.

4. Conclusion

Recently, bone and cartilage generation by autogenous cell/tissue transplantation has become one of the most promising techniques in orthopedic surgery and biomedical engineering. Several scaffold materials have been investigated for tissue engineering bone and cartilage. Hydroxyapatite (HAp) composite is an eminent one among them. It has been investigated for its clinical viability in various bone defects since the mid-1980s. Synthetic HAp exhibits good properties as a biomaterial, such as biocompatibility, bioactivity, and osteoconductivity. Therefore, it has been widely used as a bone substitute, coating on metallic implants, and scaffold for tissue engineering. HAp along with other biopolymers, ceramics, and metals produced composite scaffolds to enhance the ease of application of tissue engineering. HAp-COL and HAp-COL/HAp composite scaffolds or HAp-CNT nanocomposites for orthopedic implants are synthesized and fabricated through template method, plasma spraying, laser surface alloying, electrophoretic deposition, aerosol deposition, and a specific freeze-drying procedure. Several *in vitro* and *in vivo* experiments conducted worldwide demonstrated and proved the inevitabilities and excellences of HAp composite scaffolds in bone tissue regeneration and engineering.

Acknowledgements

The authors gratefully acknowledge the financial support by The World Academy of Sciences (TWAS) for the Research Grant No. 19-143 RG/CHE/AS_I—FR3240310168. The authors are very much grateful to Mohammad Asaduzzaman, Lecturer, Department of English, Shaheed Police Smrity College, Mirpur 14, Dhaka, Bangladesh.

Conflict of interest

The authors declare no conflict of interest.

Author details

Mohammad Shariful Islam[1*], Mohammad Abdulla-Al-Mamun[2], Alam Khan[3] and Mitsugu Todo[4]

1 Department of Veterinary and Animal Sciences, University of Rajshahi, Rajshahi, Bangladesh

2 Institute of Leather Engineering and Technology, University of Dhaka, Bangladesh

3 Department of Pharmacy, University of Rajshahi, Rajshahi, Bangladesh

4 Research Institute for Applied Mechanics, Kyushu University, Kasuga, Fukuoka, Japan

*Address all correspondence to: msips06@ru.ac.bd

References

[1] Islam MS et al. Effects of compressive ratio and sintering temperature on mechanical properties of biocompatible collagen/hydroxyapatite composite scaffolds fabricated for bone tissue engineering. Journal of Asian Ceramic Societies. 2019;7(2):183-198

[2] Gu Y, Huang W, Rahaman MN, Day DE. Bone regeneration in rat calvarial defects implanted with fibrous scaffolds composed of a mixture of silicate and borate bioactive glasses. Acta Biomaterialia. 2013;**9**:9126-9136

[3] Zhang X et al. Polymer-ceramic spiral structured scaffolds for bone tissue engineering: Effect of hydroxyapatite composition on human fetal osteoblasts. PLoS One. 2014;**9**:85871

[4] Meng J et al. Super-paramagnetic responsive nanofibrous scaffolds under static magnetic field enhance osteogenesis for bone repair in vivo. Science Reports. 2013;**3**:2655

[5] Dubok VA. Bioceramics-yesterday, today, tomorrow. Powder Metallurgy and Metal Ceramics. 2000;**39**:381-394

[6] Jarcho M. Calcium phosphate ceramics as hard tissue prosthetics. Clinical Orthopaedics and Related Research. 1981;**157**:259-278

[7] Tamai N, Myoui A, Tomita T, Nakase T, Tanaka J, Ochi T, et al. Novel hydroxyapatite ceramics with an inter connective porous structure exhibit superior osteoconduction in vivo. Journal of Biomedical Materials Research. 2002;**59A**:110-117

[8] Raquel ZL. Apatites in biological systems. Progress in Crystal Growth and Characterization. 1981;**4**:1-45.6

[9] Posner AS, Betts F. Synthetic amorphous calcium phosphate and its relation to bone mineral structure. Accounts of Chemical Research. 1975;**8**:273-281

[10] LeGeros RZ. Calcium phosphate-based osteoinductive materials. Chemical Reviews. 2008;**108**:4742-4753

[11] Habibovic P, Gbureck U, Doillon CJ, Bassett DC, van Blitterswijk CA, Barralet JE. Osteoconduction and osteoinduction of low-temperature 3D printed bioceramic implants. Biomaterials. 2008;**29**:944-953

[12] Ripamonti U, Crooks J, Khoali L, Roden L. The induction of bone formation by coral-derived calcium carbonate/hydroxyapatite constructs. Biomaterials. 2009;**30**:1428-1439

[13] Ripamonti U, Richter PW, Nilen RWN, Renton L. The induction of bone formation by smart biphasic hydroxyapatite tricalcium phosphate biomimetic matrices in the non-human primate Papio ursinus. Journal of Cellular and Molecular Medicine. 2008;**12**:1-15

[14] Yuan H, Kurashina K, de Bruijn JD, Li Y, de Groot K, Zhang X. A preliminary study on osteoinduction of two kinds of calcium phosphate ceramics. Biomaterials. 1999;**20**:1799-1806

[15] Kattimani VS et al. Hydroxyapatite-past, present, and future in bone regeneration. Bone and Tissue Regeneration Insights. 2016;7:9-19. DOI: 10.4137/BTRi.s36138

[16] Hing K, Annaz B, Saeed S, Revell P, Buckland T. Microporosity enhances bioactivity of synthetic bone graft substitutes. Journal of Materials Science. Materials in Medicine. 2005;**16**:467-475

[17] Boyde A, Corsi A, Quarto R, Cancedda R, Bianco P. Osteoconduction

in large macroporous hydroxyapatite ceramic implants: Evidence for a complementary integration and disintegration mechanism. Bone. 1999;**24**:579-589

[18] Hing KA. Bioceramic bone graft substitutes: Influence of porosity and chemistry. Clinical Orthopaedics and Related Research. 2005;**2**:184-199

[19] Hench LL, Wilson J. Surface-active biomaterials. Science. 1984;**226**:630-706

[20] Hulbert SF, Young FA, Mathews RS, Klawitter JJ, Talbert CD, Stelling FH. Potential of ceramic materials as permanently implantable skeletal prostheses. Journal of Biomedical Materials Research. Part A. 1970;**4**:433-456

[21] Mobasherpour I, Hashjin MS, Toosi SSR, Kamachali RD. Effect of the addition ZrO2-Al2O3 on nanocrystalline hydroxyapatite bending strength and fracture toughness. Ceramics International. 2009;**35**:1569-1574

[22] Thomson RC, Wake MC, Yaszemski MJ, Mikos AG. Biodegradable polymer scaffolds to regenerate organs. Advances in Polymer Science. 1997;**122**:245-274

[23] Persidis A. Tissue engineering. Nature Biotechnology. 1999;**17**(5):508-510

[24] Service RF. Tissue engineers build new bone. Science. 2000;**289**(5484):1498-1500

[25] Petite H, Viateau V, Bensaid W, Meunier A, de Pollak C, Bourguignon M, et al. Tissue engineered bone regeneration. Nature Biotechnology. 2000;**18**(9):959-963

[26] Azevedo MC, Reis RL, Claase MB, Grijpma DW, Feijen J. Development and properties of polycaprolactone/hydroxyapatite composite biomaterials. Journal of Materials Science. Materials in Medicine. 2003;**14**:103-107

[27] Guarino V, Causa F, Netti PA, Ciapetti G, Pagani S, Martini D, et al. The role of hydroxyapatite as solid signal on performance of PCL porous scaffolds for bone tissue regeneration. Journal of Biomedical Materials Research Part B: Applied Biomaterials. 2008;**86**:548-557

[28] Kim HW, Knowles JC, Kim HE. Hydroxyapatite/poly(εcaprolactone) composite coatings on hydroxyapatite porous bone scaffold for drug delivery. Biomaterials. 2004;**25**:1279-1287

[29] Mourinño V, Boccaccini AR. Bone tissue engineering therapeutics-controlled drug delivery in three dimensional scaffolds. Journal of the Royal Society, Interface. 2010;**7**: 209-227

[30] Kim SS et al. Poly(lactide-co-glycolide)/hydroxyapatite composite scaffolds for bone tissue engineering. Biomaterials. 2006;**27**:1399-1409

[31] Islam MS, Todo M. Effects of sintering temperature on the compressive mechanical properties of collagen/hydroxyapatite composite scaffolds for bone tissue engineering. Materials Letters. 2016;**173**:231-234

[32] Balani K, Zhang T, Karakoti A, Li WZ, Seal S, Agarwal A. In situ carbon nanotube reinforcements in a plasma-sprayed aluminum oxide nanocomposite coating. Acta Materialia. 2008;**56**:571-579

[33] Ma RZ, Wu J, Wei BQ, Liang J, Wu DH. Processing and properties of carbon nanotubes-nano-SiC ceramic. Journal of Materials Science. 1998;**33**:5243-5246

[34] Lahiri D, Singh V, Keshri AK, Seal S, Agarwal A. Carbon nanotube toughened hydroxyapatite by spark plasma

sintering: Microstructural evolution and multiscale tribological properties. Carbon N Y. 2010;**48**:3103-3120

[35] Cheng GJ, Pirzada D, Cai M, Mohanty P, Bandyopadhyay A. Bioceramic coating of hydroxyapatite on titanium substrate with Nd-YAG laser. Materials Science and Engineering: C. 2005;**25**:541-547

[36] Singh I, Kaya C, Shaffer MSP, Thomas BC, Boccaccini AR. Bioactive ceramic coatings containing carbon nanotubes on metallic substrates by electrophoretic deposition. Journal of Materials Science. 2006;**41**:8144-8151

[37] Hahn B, Lee J, Park D, et al. Mechanical and in vitro biological performances of hydroxyapatite–carbon nanotube composite coatings deposited on Ti by aerosol deposition. Acta Biomaterialia. 2009;**5**:3205-3214

[38] Li A, Sun K, Dong W, Zhao D. Mechanical properties, microstructure and histocompatibility of MWCNTs/HAp biocomposites. Materials Letters. 2007;**61**:1839-1844

[39] Li H, Zhao N, Liu Y, et al. Fabrication and properties of carbon nanotubes reinforced Fe/hydroxyapatite composites by in situ chemical vapor deposition. Composites Part A: Applied Science and Manufacturing. 2008;**39**:1128-1132

[40] Omori M, Okubo A, Otsubo M, Hashida T, Tohji K. Consolidation of multiwalled carbon nanotube and hydroxyapatite coating by the spark plasma system (SPS). Key Engineering Materials. 2004;**25**(4-256):395-398

[41] Xu JL, Khor KA, Sui JJ, Chen WN. Preparation and characterization of a novel hydroxyapatite/carbon nanotubes composite and its interaction with osteoblastlike cells. Materials Science and Engineering: C. 2009;**29**:44-49

[42] Phanny Y. Development and characterization of polymer/bioceramic composite porous biomaterials for bone tissue engineering [thesis]. Japan: Kyushu University; 2014

[43] Catherine G, Charles JD. Facilitating tissue infiltration and angiogenesis in a tubular collagen scaffold. Journal of Biomedical Materials Research Part A. 2009;**93**:615-624. DOI: 10.1002/jbm.a.32568

[44] Heinemann C, Heinemann S, Bernhardt A, Worch H, Hanke T. Novel textile chitosan scaffolds promote spreading, proliferation, and differentiation of osteoblasts. Biomacromolecules. 2008;**9**:2913-2920. DOI: 10.1021/bm800693d

[45] Girotto D, Urbani S, Brun P, Renier D, Barbucci R, Abatangelo G. Tissue-specific gene expression in chondrocytes grown on three-dimensional hyaluronic acid scaffolds. Biomaterials. 2003;**24**:3265-3275. DOI: 10.1016/S0142-9612(03)00160-1

[46] Park JE, Todo M. Development and characterization of reinforced poly(l-lactide) scaffolds for bone tissue engineering. Journal of Materials Science. Materials in Medicine. 2011;**22**:1171-1182. DOI: 10.1007/s10856-011-4289-4

[47] Joshua RP, Andrew H, Ketul CP. Biodegradable poly(ε-caprolactone) nanowires for bone tissue engineering applications. Biomaterials. 2009;**30**:780-788. DOI: 10.1016/j.biomaterials.2008.10.022

[48] Lohan A, Marzahn U, El Sayed K, Haisch A, Kohl B, Müller RD, et al. In vitro and in vivo neo-cartilage formation by heterotopic chondrocytes seeded on PGA scaffolds. Histochemistry and Cell Biology. 2011;**136**:57-69. DOI: 10.1007/s00418-011-0822-2

[49] Wiria FE, Chua CK, Leong KF, Quah ZY, Chandrasekaran M, Lee MW. Improved biocomposite development of poly(vinyl alcohol) and hydroxyapatite for tissue engineering scaffold fabrication using selective laser sintering. Journal of Materials Science. Materials in Medicine. 2008;**19**:989-996. DOI: 10.1007/s10856-007-3176-5

[50] Zhang X, Guo YLi DX, Wang R, Fan HS, Xiao YM, Zhang L, et al. The effect of loading icariin on biocompatibility and bioactivity of porous β-TCP ceramic. Journal of Materials Science: Materials in Medicine. 2011;**22**:371-379. DOI: 10.1007/s10856-010-4198-y

[51] Udoh KMunar ML, Maruta M, Matsuya S, Ishikawa K. Effects of sintering temperature on physical and compositional properties of α-tricalcium phosphate foam. Dental Materials Journal. 2010;**29**:154-159

[52] Arpornmaeklong P, Pripatnanont P, Suwatwirote N. Properties of chitosan-collagen sponges and osteogenic differentiation of rat-bone-marrow stromal cells. International Journal of Oral and Maxillofacial Surgery. 2008;**37**:357-366. DOI: 10.1016/j.ijom.2007.11.014

[53] Akkouch A, Zhang Z, Rouabhia M. A novel collagen/hydroxyapatite/poly(lactide-co-ε-caprolactone) biodegradable and bioactive 3D porous scaffold for bone regeneration. Journal of Biomedical Materials Research Part A. 2011;**96**:693-704. DOI: 10.1002/jbm.a.33033

[54] Salerno A, Zeppetelli S, Di Maio E, Iannace S. Processing/structure/property relationship of multi-scaled PCL and PCL-HA composite scaffolds prepared via gas foaming and NaCl reverse templating. Biotechnology and Bioengineering. 2011;**108**:963-976. DOI: 10.1002/bit.23018

[55] Hiraoka Y, Kimura Y, Ueda H, Tabata Y. Fabrication and biocompatibility of collagen sponge reinforced with poly(glycolic acid) fiber. Tissue Engineering. 2003;**9**:1101-1112. DOI: 10.1089/10763270360728017

[56] Wahl DA, Czernuszka JT. Collagen-hydroxyapatite composites for hard tissue repair. European Cells & Materials. 2006;**11**:43-56

[57] Du C, Cui FZ, Zhu XD, de Groot K. Three dimensional nano-HAp/collagen matrix loading with osteogenic cells in organ culture. Journal of Biomedical Materials Research. 1999;**44**:407-415

[58] Clarke KI, Graves SE, Wong ATC, Triffitt JT, Francis MJO, Czernuszka JT. Investigation into the formation and mechanical-properties of a bioactive material based on collagen and calcium-phosphate. Journal of Materials Science. Materials in Medicine. 1993;**4**:107-110

[59] Wu TJ, Huang HH, Lan CW, Lin CH, Hsu FY, Wang YJ. Studies on the microspheres comprised of reconstituted collagen and hydroxyapatite. Biomaterials. 2004;**25**:651-658

[60] Wang X, Grogan SP, Rieser F, Winkelmann V, Maquet V, Berge ML, et al. Tissue engineering of biphasic cartilage constructs using various biodegradable scaffolds: An in vitro study. Biomaterials. 2004;**25**:3681-3688

[61] Rovira A, Amedee J, Bareille R, Rabaud M. Colonization of a calcium phosphate elastin-solubilized peptide-collagen composite material by human osteoblasts. Biomaterials. 1996;**17**:1535-1540

[62] Cai L, Wang Q, Gu C, Wu J, Wang J, Kang N, et al. Vascular and micro-environmental influences on MSC-coral hydroxyapatite construct-based bone tissue engineering. Biomaterials. 2011;**32**:8497-8505

[63] Kikuchi M, Itoh S, Ichinose S, Shinomiya K, Tanaka J. Self-organization mechanism in a bone-like hydroxyapatite/collagen nanocomposite synthesized in vitro and its biological reaction in vivo. Biomaterials. 2001;**22**:1705-1711

[64] Sotome S, Uemura T, Kikuchi M, Chen J, Itoh S, Tanaka J, et al. Synthesis and in vivo evaluation of a novel hydroxyapatite/collagenalginate as a bone filler and a drug delivery carrier of bone morphogenetic protein. Materials Science and Engineering: C. 2004;**24**:341-347

[65] Ripamonti U, Roden LC, Renton LF. Osteoinductive hydroxyapatite-coated titanium implants. Biomaterials. 2012;**33**(15):3813-3823

[66] Caria PH, Kawachi EY, Bertran CA, Camilli JA. Biological assessment porousimplant hydroxyapatite of combined with periosteal grafting in maxillary defects. Journal of Oral and Maxillofacial Surgery. 2007;**65**:847-854

[67] Okazaki M, Ohmae H, Takahashi J, Kimura H, Sakuda M. Insolubilized properties of UV-irradiated C03 apatite-collagen composites. Biomaterials. 1990;**11**:568-572

[68] Du C, Cui FZ, Zhang W, Feng QL, Zhu XD, de Groot K. Formation of calcium phosphate/collagen composites through mineralization of collagen matrix. Journal of Biomedical Materials Research. 2000;**50**:518-527

[69] Kikuchi M, Itoh S, Ichinose S, Shinomiya K, Tanaka J. Self-organization mechanism in a bone-like hydroxyapatite/collagen nanocomposite synthesized in vitro and its biological reaction in vivo. Biomaterials. 2001;**22**:1705-1711

[70] Itoh S, Kikuchi M, Koyama Y, Takakuda K, Shinomiya K, Tanaka J. Development of an artificial vertebral body using a novel biomaterial, hydroxyapatite/collagen composite. Biomaterials. 2002;**23**:3919-3926

[71] Yamasaki Y, Yoshida Y, Okazaki M, Shimazu A, Kubo T, Akagawa Y, et al. Action of FGMgCO3Apcollagen composite in promoting bone formation. Biomaterials. 2003;**24**:4913-4920

[72] Martins VCA, Goissis G. Nonstoichiometric hydroxyapatite: Anionic collagen composite as a support for the double sustained release of gentamicin and norfloxacin/ciprofloxacin. Artificial Organs. 2000;**24**:224-230

[73] Suh H, Han D-W, Park J-C, Lee DH, Lee WS, Han CD. A bone replaceable artificial bone substitute: Osteoinduction by combining with bone inducing agent. Artificial Organs. 2001;**25**:459-466

Section 2

Medical Materials

Chapter 4

Development of New Advanced Ti-Mo Alloys for Medical Applications

Petrică Vizureanu, Mădălina Simona Bălţatu and Andrei Victor Sandu

Abstract

The use of titanium and titanium-based alloys with applications in implantology and dentistry has made remarkable progress in the promotion of new technologies and new materials that have been developed in recent years. This is justified thanks to their excellent mechanical, physical, and biological performance. Today's generation promotes new titanium alloys, with nontoxic elements and long-term performance and without rejection of the human body. This book chapter describes new original compositions of Ti-based alloys for medical applications, with improved properties compared to existing classical alloys (C.p. Ti, Ti6Al4V, CoCrMo, etc.). The addition of nontoxic elements such as Mo, Si, Zr, and Ta brings benefits as reduced modulus of elasticity, increased corrosion resistance, and improved biocompatibility.

Keywords: Ti-Mo alloys, microstructural characterization, corrosion resistance, low elastic modulus

1. Introduction

Materials with the possibility of performing a biological function are increasingly sought. In the medical field, implants require a high compatibility with the hard tissue for osteointegration and bone formation and a compatibility with the soft tissue for the adhesion of the epithelium to them and the acquisition of antibacterial properties for inhibiting or forming the biofilm at the interface. These biofunctional characteristics have two contradictory properties: inhibition and enhancement of protein adsorption, respectively, and cell adhesion [1, 2].

The usual classification of synthetic biomaterials is carried out structurally, according to the classes of materials used. The main types of synthetic biomaterials are metallic, ceramic, polymeric, composite, and of natural origin, but they can also be divided into several categories, as can be seen in **Figure 1**.

Biocompatible materials are intended to "work under biological constraint" and thereby become adapted to various medical applications.

When a metallic material is implanted in a human body, immediate reactions occur between their surface and the living tissues. In other words, an immediate reaction during the introduction period is determined and defines the biofunctionality of the metallic material [3].

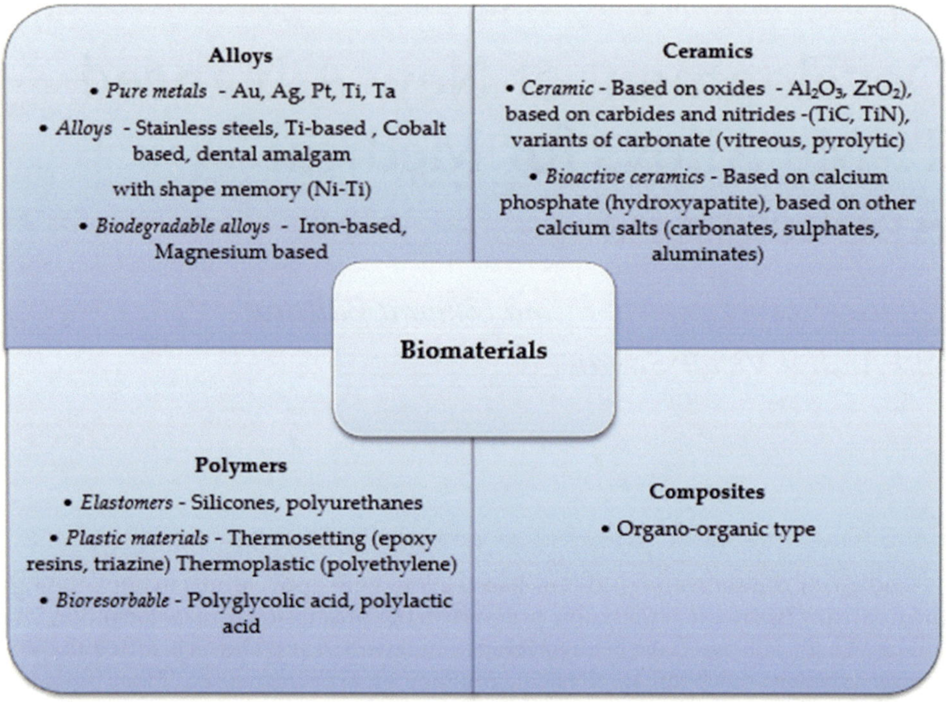

Figure 1.
The main types of biomaterials [4].

The quality of a material used in the construction of an implant must respect the following two criteria: the biochemical criterion and the biomechanical criterion. According to the biochemical criterion, the applicability of a material is determined by its biocompatibility, and from the biomechanical point of view of fatigue resistance, it is the most important parameter but not the only one.

The most used metallic biomaterials are stainless steels, Co-Cr alloys, titanium alloys, and magnesium-based alloys. Each class of biomaterials has its advantages and disadvantages (**Figure 2**), their use in the execution of different implants being influenced by both the properties of the biomaterials and the functional requirements imposed to the implants [5].

Among the most important factors that intervene on a biomaterial successfully integrated in the human body, we mention the physical-chemical properties, the design, the biocompatibility, the surgical technique applied to the implantation, and last but not least, the patient's health.

The selection of materials used in contact with living cells or tissues for implantation in the human body, as biomaterials, is determined primarily by their acceptance by the human tissues with which they interact (biocompatibility) and by the ability to perform their functional role for which they were implanted (biofunctionality) [6].

Out of the metallic biomaterials, a special interest is for those with osteotropic structure, of which the titanium belongs. These biomaterials, thanks to the chemical and micromorphological biocompatibility with the bone tissue, achieve with this physical-chemical connection, the interface phenomenon being assimilated with the linking osteogenesis.

Titanium alloys are frequently used, due to the need of replacing stainless steels and cobalt-based alloys that have limitations in use, causing some deficiencies of biocompatibility with human tissues. These deficiencies are caused by some elements present in their chemical composition (e.g., nickel), which have a toxic effect

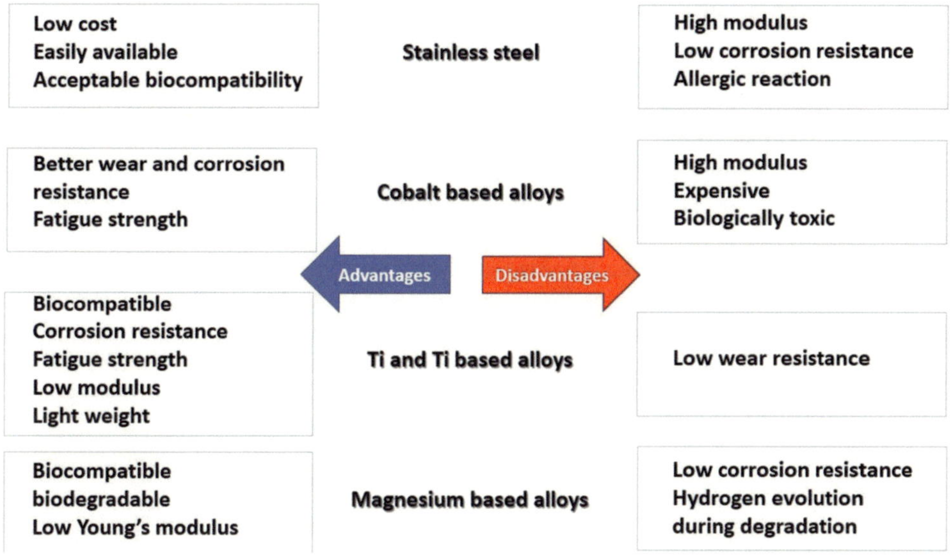

Figure 2.
Main characteristics of metallic orthopedic implants [6].

on human tissues, causing inflammatory allergic reactions or implant rejection reactions [7].

The properties of the titanium are as follows:

- melting point—the titanium melts at 1660°, and it can be sterilized without risk at 300°;
- resistance—the implants are made from a single pure titanium bar by mechanical processing, giving them maximum resistance;
- hardness—the titanium has a hardness comparable to that of steel, giving it special mechanical quality;
- rigidity—the implants do not deform when applying, mounting, or milling forces nor in the biomechanics of chewing;
- nonmagnetic—the titanium has no magnetic effect, resulting in good tissue supportability;
- regenerative and therapeutic action—research and practical experience have highlighted the healing qualities of titanium oxide;
- neutral pH—titanium dioxide, TiO_2, which is formed immediately around the metal molecules, has a pH of 7, completely neutral;
- biological immunity—the implant can be stimulated in contact with the bone, surrounding tissues and the oral cavity environment;
- excellent resistance to electric shock—the titanium has a very low thermal conductivity; and
- light weight—the density of titanium is close to that of light alloys [4, 8].

The biocompatibility of titanium is a consequence of the presence of the superficial oxide layer. The chemical properties and therefore the chemical processes on the interface are determined precisely by this layer of oxide and not by the metal itself. This feature is applicable to all metal materials used in the manufacturing of implants and prosthetic parts. Among the metal materials used for hard tissue repair in human body, the elastic modulus of titanium (about 80–110 GPa) is the closest to hard human tissue, which can reduce the mechanical incompatibility between metal implants and bone tissue [9].

Titanium alloys are used for medical applications in multiple fields in human body and became the first choice for orthopedic products. **Figure 3** shows the main applications of titanium alloys used in orthopedic applications [2–8].

In conclusion, it can be said that titanium biomaterials, by its properties, respond to almost all the requirements necessary for the achievement of osteogenesis, osteointegration, and durability over time. The pure titanium implant offers perfect compatibility, correct and concrete osteogenesis, and demonstrable time-lapse viability.

Adding the alloying elements gives titanium a wide range of properties through different microstructures and properties.

After microstructure, the alloys are grouped into three categories depending on the type of stabilizing elements added to the titanium alloy. The mechanical properties and corrosion resistance of the alloys depend on the morphology and structure of the α or β phase particles in the alloy matrix.

Thus, the alloying elements are divided into three categories as follows:

- α stabilizers: C, N_2, O_2, and Al;
- β stabilizers: V, Nb, Mo, Ta, Fe, Mn, Cr, Co, W, Ni, Cu, Si, and H_2; and
- neutral elements: Zr, Sn, Hf, Ge, and Th [1, 5, 8].

Over the years, many titanium alloys have been developed and investigated for the implantation of implants for medical applications, of which few have been accepted by the human body, namely those that have certain properties necessary for long-term success.

The biocompatibility of an alloy depends on the alloying elements. Alloying elements such as Zr, Ta, Nb, and Sn do not affect cell viability and have shown a reduced amount of ions released into the body, but Al and V contribute to reducing cell viability. Other elements such as Ag, Co, Cr, and Cu have moderate cytotoxic behavior, but their presence in these alloys significantly reduces their toxicity [1–5]. By analyzing the current research, these alloys were studied in order to develop

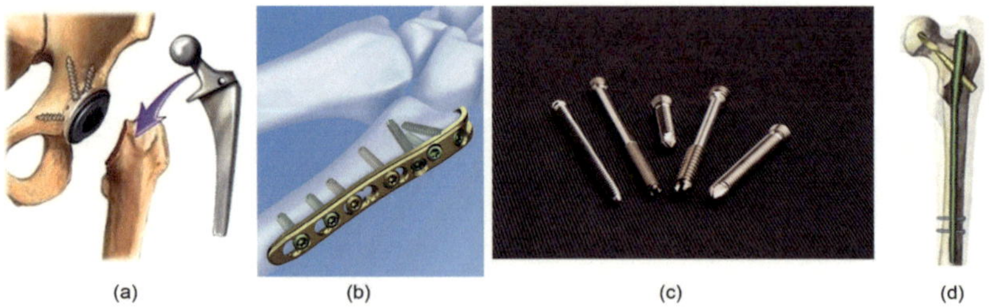

Figure 3.
Orthopedic products made by titanium and titanium alloys: (a) endoprosthesis for joint replacement; (b) system plate screws for bone fracture repair; (c) screws for bone repair; and (d) intramedullary nail [2, 9].

new recipes of titanium-based alloys with elements with high biocompatibility on human tissue such as Mo, Ta, Zr, and Si [10, 11].

2. Characterization of the obtained titanium alloys

The experimental tests aim at a characterization of new developed titanium alloys by chemical, structural, surface, and mechanical analyses.

This chapter describes the following investigations for the new alloys developed:

- **Development of alloys** was carried out using a Vacuum Arc Remelting installation for the elaboration of homogeneous alloys.
- **Elemental composition** is necessary to determine the percentages of the chemical elements that make up the elaborated titanium alloys.
- **Structural characterization** is necessary for the study of the microstructure, the crystallographic orientation, the texture, and the identification of the constituent phases.
- **Mechanical characterization** highlights the mechanical properties of the developed titanium alloys: hardness and elasticity module.
- **Corrosion resistance** determines the stability of the proposed alloys in the simulated body fluids.
- **Surface characterization** takes into account the measurement of the contact angle of the surface of the alloys for achieving/optimizing the adhesion and cell proliferation.

2.1 Vacuum arc remelting

In order to obtain the titanium alloys, the MRF ABJ 900 Vacuum Arc Remelting has been used. Vacuum arc remelting is a commonly used process in the development of alloys. The process itself is used to refill the ingots and refine the structure by using nonconsumable mobile electrode of thorium tungsten. The process itself can also be used to obtain special alloys, superalloys, and titanium alloys.

In principle, the process of remelting with a vacuum arc is a process based on continuous melting with the use of the electric arc and nonconsumable mobile electrode.

Advantages of using this equipment are as follows:

- It can achieve very high melting temperatures.
- It ensures the possibility of melting the metallic vacuum samples under a protective atmosphere by means of a nonconsumable mobile electrode of thorium tungsten.
- It creates alloys with uniform composition, through repeated remeltings.
- It ensures the possibility of mixing elements with different melting temperatures.

- It can use various crucibles for elaboration and ensure the possibility of obtaining the samples under specific conditions in the form of a pill of different shapes and sizes.

- Loading and unloading is done in a simple way by lifting the cover that is caught in the hinge to the rest of the camera.

- It is illuminated with a halogen lamp, thus helping to control the melting of the alloying elements in the process [12].

Figure 4 shows all stages of titanium alloying, which includes the weighing of the raw material, the loading of the alloying elements, and the final semi-finished obtained products.

The load calculation has considered the characteristics of the different alloying elements and their physical-chemical properties.

Elaboration of the alloys was carried out in two charges to obtain two alloys in each charge. **Table 1** shows alloys proposed the cavities used for each alloy.

Elaboration of the titanium alloys made with a vacuum arc melting system, took place by the melting of the elements, and followed by the remeltings of alloys for six times, a necessary operation for the refining and homogenization of the alloys. The melting of the elements took place uniformly, resulting alloys with a precise and homogeneous chemical composition. The samples had a homogeneous structure, which means that the installation, the elaboration protocol, and the elements were chosen correctly.

After the solidification, two samples of each alloy were obtained in the form of ingots, shapes, and different masses but with sufficient quantity for taking the specimens required for all proposed laboratory tests.

2.2 Determination of the chemical composition of titanium alloys by EDAX analysis

A complete characterization of a metallic material consists in knowing its composition, the concentration of the various elements, or the impurities in the mass of the alloy. An extremely important aspect is the determination as precisely as possible of the chemical composition of the titanium alloys obtained after elaboration.

The EDAX system is a microanalysis detector, equipped with an electron microscope, which uses the resulting X-ray energy on the surface of the samples.

Determination of chemical composition can be performed, both punctually and in a well-defined region on the surface of the analyzed sample.

This method is a variant of X-ray fluorescence spectroscopy, in which the sample investigation is based on the interactions between the electromagnetic radiation and the sample, analyzing the X radiation emitted by the sample as a response to the charging of particles loaded with electric charges. The characterization possibilities are largely according to the fundamental principle that each chemical element has a unique atomic structure that allows the characteristic X-rays of the atomic structure of an element to characterize it uniquely from another.

In order to achieve the structural and thermal characterization, it is necessary to identify the chemical composition of the alloys obtained. EDAX microanalysis with energy dispersion of X radiation was used to determine the chemical composition of the TiMo alloys developed. Determination of the chemical composition by EDAX microanalysis is the first laboratory investigation required to highlight the proportions obtained between the pure chemical elements and was performed on titanium alloys obtained.

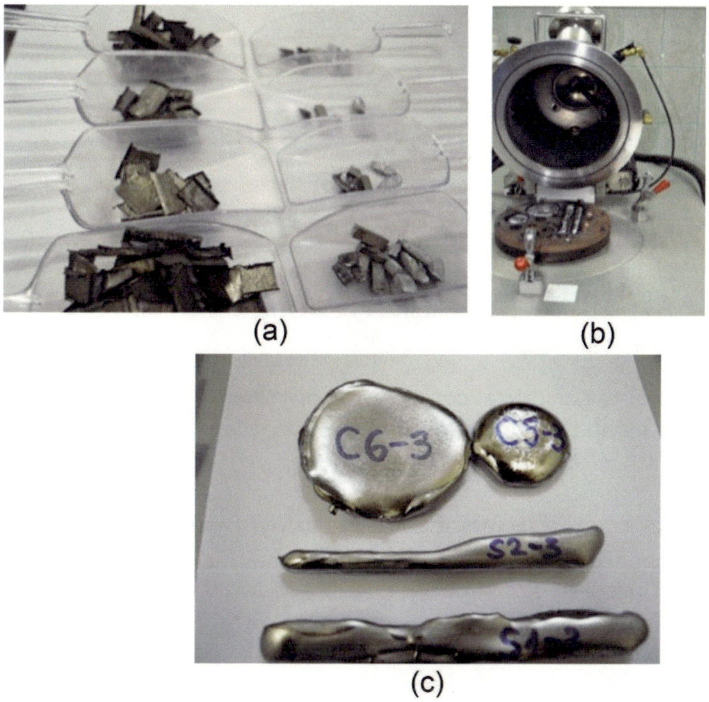

Figure 4.
Stages of titanium alloying obtaining process: (a) weighing of raw materials and gravimetric dosing; (b) loading of the raw material; and (c) titanium semi-products obtained after solidification [12].

Alloy element	Ti	Mo	Si	Zr	Ta
			(% weight)		
Ti15Mo0.5Si	84.50	15.00	0.50	—	—
Ti20Mo0.5Si	79.50	20.00	0.50	—	—
Ti15Mo7Zr10Ta	68.00	15.00	—	7.00	10.00
Ti20Mo7Zr10Ta	63.00	20.00	—	7.00	10.00

Table 1.
Chemical composition proposed of the new titanium alloys.

In order to validate the results regarding the concentration, for each sample, 10 measurements on five different areas were done.

To determine the chemical composition of the obtained titanium alloys, the Vega Tescan LMH II equipment was performed using the EDAX by Bruker attached to the SEM equipment.

For the determination of the chemical composition of alloys obtained from the TiMo system, samples having dimensions of 10 mm × 10 mm × 5 mm were used. Before being examined, the samples were ground on abrasive paper to remove impurities and titanium oxide film on the surface of the alloy.

Table 2 shows the mass percentages of the elements identified in the alloy composition, the percentages of the elements varying slightly with the theoretical batch calculation.

Figures 5–8 highlight EDX spectrum and element mapping of titanium alloys.

Alloy element	Ti	Mo	Si	Zr	Ta
			(% weight)		
Ti15Mo0.5Si	79.28	19.95	0.77	—	—
Ti20Mo0.5Si	78.98	20.06	0.96	—	—
Ti15Mo7Zr10Ta	75.40	10.41	—	7.69	6.50
Ti20Mo7Zr10Ta	71.51	14.05	—	7.04	7.40

Table 2.
Chemical compositions of titanium alloys, expressed as a mass percentage, according to the EDX measurements.

The analysis of the chemical composition obtained revealed that the main elements identified in the alloys elaborated are Ti, Mo, Zr, Ta, and Si, without the presence of other inclusions.

2.3 Structural characterization of titanium alloys by optical microscopy

Microscopic methods of structural analysis are used to characterize the materials based on their structure, constituents and phases present (nature, shape, dimensions, and distribution), and possible structural defects (pores, cracks, structural inhomogeneities, etc.). Structural analysis was performed using the OPTIKA XDS-3 MET microscope.

In order to investigate the metallographic structure, the preparation of the metallographic samples of the experimental titanium alloys included a sequence of steps: cutting to appropriate dimensions (e.g., 10 mm × 10 mm × 5 mm), incorporation in epoxy resin, grinding and polishing, and chemical attack with specific reagents (a solution with 10 mL of HF, 5 mL of HNO_3, and 85 mL of H_2O) for 30 s. After the preparation of the samples, this was analyzed at the optical microscope at various magnification powers in order to obtain detailed images on the microstructure.

Figure 9 highlights images obtained by optical microscopy for titanium alloys at 100× magnification.

In **Figure 9**, the structure of titanium alloys with aspects of the specific grains of titanium is presented. The images obtained by optical microscopy for the elaborated alloys show a dendritic structure with irregular grain boundaries. These coarse structures are specific to β alloys.

The variation of the α, α + β, and β type phases consists of the differences in chemical composition of the constituent elements. The high percentage of β-stabilizing elements (Mo, Ta, and Si) led to the formation of a β-type structure, very well highlighted in the elaborated TiMo alloys.

2.4 Mechanical characterization

2.4.1 Microindentation method

The measurement of the longitudinal elastic modulus for the obtained titanium alloys was achieved by the microindentation method. This method consists of penetrating the surface of the sample with a conical palpate at a certain force.

From a practical point of view, the indentation characterization presents a major advantage over the standard methods of testing on standardized tests, namely, the testing can be done directly on the finished pieces.

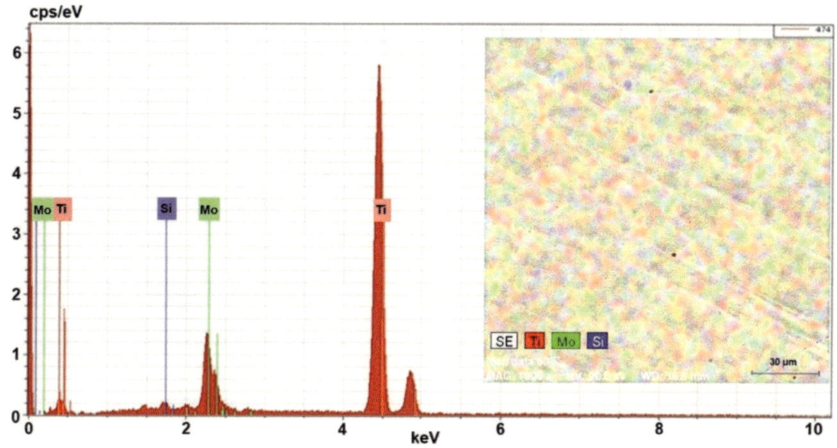

Figure 5.
EDX spectrum and mapping for Ti15Mo0.50Si alloy.

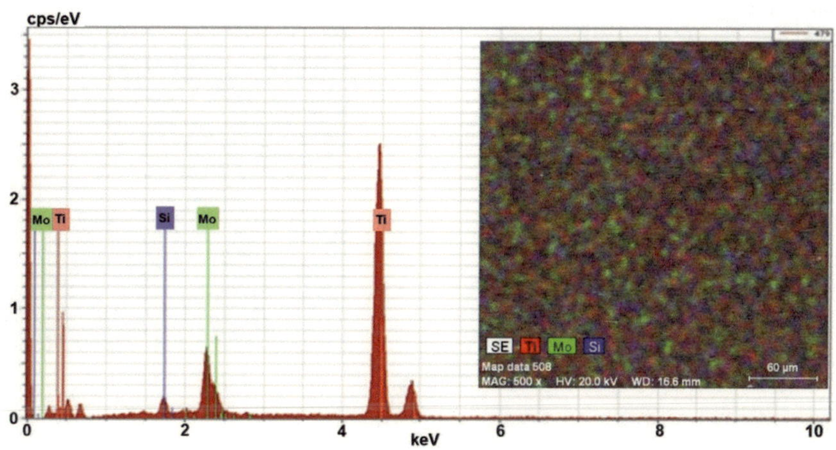

Figure 6.
EDX spectrum and mapping for Ti20Mo0.50Si alloy.

During the microindentation test, the values of the loading forces are recorded relative to the penetration depth of the indenter in the material. Based on the loading-unloading curve, a number of sizes can be determined that allow the characterization of the materials.

Figure 10 shows the response of the alloys during the indentation tests in the form of force-depth dependencies. The values of the modulus of elasticity for the titanium alloys resulting from the indentation test are shown in **Table 3**.

Among the mechanical properties that are considered when evaluating a biomaterial is the longitudinal elasticity module. If the biomaterial is used for orthopedic implants, it must have a modulus of longitudinal elasticity equivalent to that of the bone, which varies between 4 and 30 GPa, depending on the type of bone and the direction of measurement [13–15].

A low modulus is reliable in inhibiting the bone resorption and enhancing the remodeling of bones, which may be due to the excellent stress transmission between the bone and the implant. A biomedical orthopedic implant should have a Young modulus matching or closer to that of human bone to avoid the stress shielding effect.

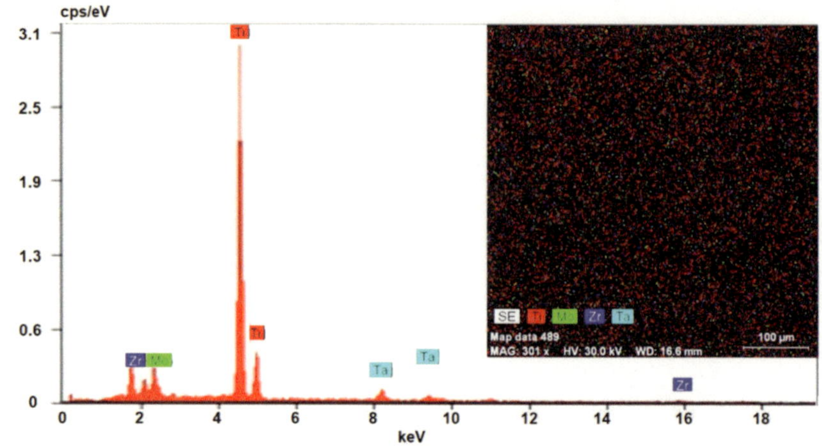

Figure 7.
EDX spectrum and mapping for Ti15Mo7Zr10Ta alloy.

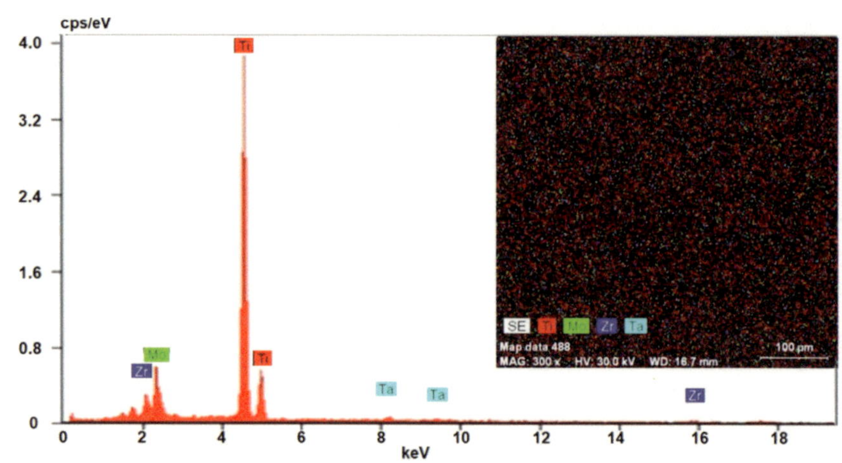

Figure 8.
EDX spectrum and mapping for Ti20Mo7Zr10Ta alloy.

The developed titanium alloys have a low modulus of elasticity, close to that of the bone, with the exception of the Ti15Mo7Zr10Ta alloy and significantly lower values than CoCr alloys.

If the balance between mechanical properties and biocompatibility is achieved by both the implant and the bone tissue, the risk of negative effects is very small. The use of titanium materials with a low modulus of elasticity seems to be a good solution, and the chances of using the material for medical purposes are increasing.

2.4.2 Determination of hardness for titanium alloys

Hardness is a property of materials that express their ability to resist the action of mechanically penetrating a tougher body into its surface. When determining the hardness of the materials, the size of the traces produced by a penetration body, characterized by a certain shape and size, and the force acting on it is taken into account.

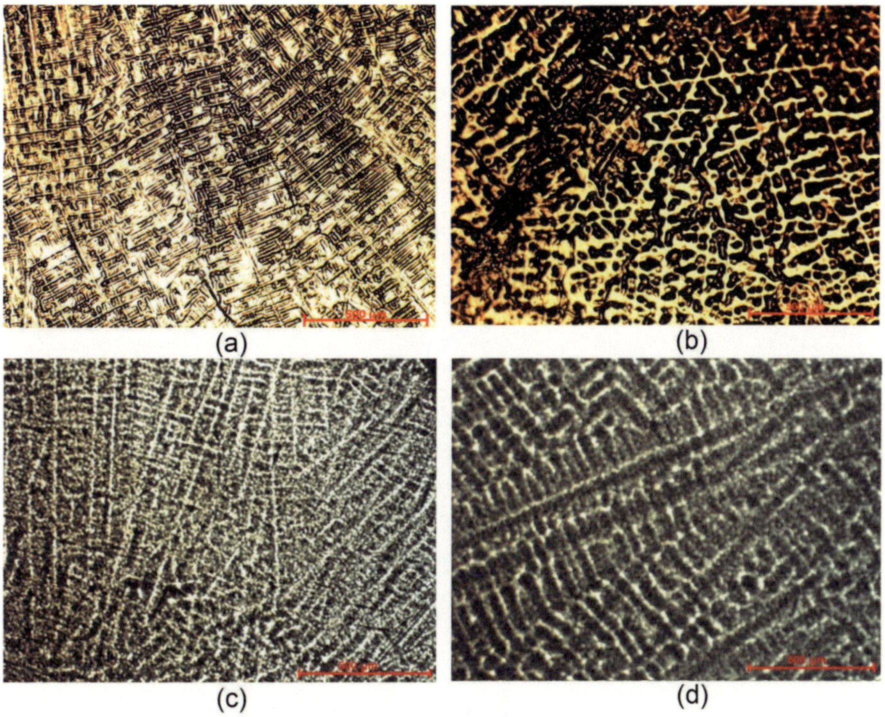

Figure 9.
Optical microstructure of alloys investigated at 100× magnification power: (a) Ti15Mo0.5Si, (b) Ti20Mo0.5Si, (c) Ti15Mo7Zr10Ta, and (d) Ti20Mo7Zr10Ta.

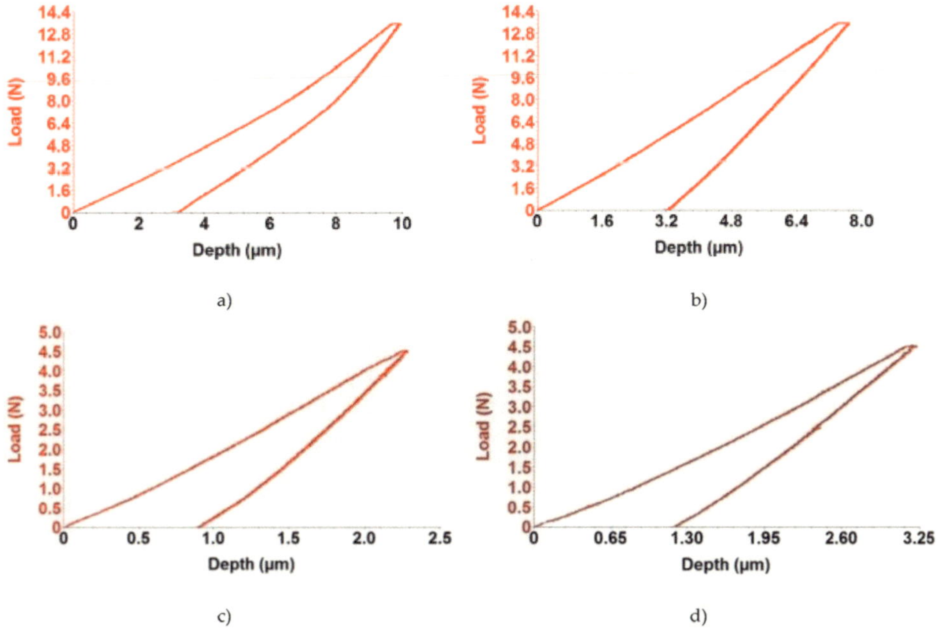

Figure 10.
The force-depth curve of the micro-indentation test for the investigated alloys: (a) Ti15Mo0.5Si, (b) Ti20Mo0.5Si, (c) Ti15Mo7Zr10Ta, and (d) Ti20Mo7Zr10Ta.

Alloy	Ti15Mo0.5Si	Ti20Mo0.5Si	Ti15Mo7Zr10Ta	Ti20Mo7Zr10Ta	C.p. Ti	Ti6Al4V	CoCr alloys	Human bone
Elastic modulus (GPa)	19.81	37.53	76.88	43.41	**105**	**110**	**240**	**17**

The bold values represent the values of the classical alloys used in implantology, values that do not belong to us and are for a comparative points. They were bold to see the good results of our alloys.

Table 3.
Elastic modulus values for titanium alloys measured by indentation test [13, 14, 16, 17].

The methods for determining the hardness, depending on the speed of the force on the penetrator, are classified into static methods, where the drive speed is below 1 mm/s, and dynamic methods for which the drive speed exceeds this value.

The Vickers hardness determination method uses a diamond penetrator in the form of a pyramid with a square base and consists in pressing it at a reduced speed and with a certain predetermined force F on the surface of the test material. The Vickers hardness, symbolized by HV, is expressed by the ratio of the applied force F to the area of the lateral surface of the residual trace produced by the penetrator. The trace is considered to be a straight pyramid with a square base, with diagonal d, having the same angle as the penetrator at the top.

For the Vickers hardness determination method, at least three attempts are made on the test material. For each trace, the average diagonal value is calculated based on the magnitude of the two diagonals measured. It is recognized that the difference in diagonal dimensions is within an error margin of not more than 2%.

The hardness measurements highlight resistance and provide information on the behavior of the studied materials. In this way, we can analyze titanium alloys developed for the purpose of fitting them into a specific medical application (**Table 4**).

HV hardness measurements on titanium alloys were performed with Wilson Wolpert 751N.

Both systems studied have different hardness results. Compared to other titanium biomaterials, TMZT alloys have a higher hardness, but close to the Ti6Al4V alloy, which are most commonly used in implantology. An important aspect that might have contributed to the increased hardness is the amount of stabilizing β elements. It can be observed that as the amount of stabilizing β elements increases (Mo and Ta), it decreases the hardness values.

2.5 Corrosion resistance

Corrosion represents the physical-chemical, spontaneous, reversible, and undesirable destruction of metals and alloys under the chemical, electrochemical, or biological action of the environment.

Corrosion monitoring is the practice of qualitative assessment and quantitative measurement of the corrosivity of an environment on a metal or an alloy immersed in this environment. Monitoring tests can be performed using mechanical, electrical, electrochemical, or chemical methods [18–20]. The nature of the monitoring sensor depends on the technique chosen for the study, the purpose pursued, and the particular characteristics of the sample used. In the older methods, the electrical measurements were often used, the monitoring technique and the methods of processing the experimental data being generally very laborious. The advances in the field of microelectronics have allowed the signals of the electrochemical sensors to be strictly conditioned, appropriately amplified, and processed based on complex data processing programs.

Some techniques and methods of measurement allow continuous monitoring of corrosion—the sample is permanently exposed in the corrosion environment, while the discontinuous methods are done only in specialized laboratories.

Alloy	Ti15Mo0.5Si	Ti20Mo0.5Si	Ti15Mo7Zr10Ta	Ti20Mo7Zr10Ta	C.P. Ti	Ti6Al4V	CoCr alloys
HV	233.37	165.18	462.33	321.31	**128**	**381**	**600**

The bold values represent the values of the classical alloys used in implantology, values that do not belong to us and are for a comparative points. They were bold to see the good results of our alloys.

Table 4.
The hardness values of titanium alloys measured by the Vickers method [5, 13, 14].

Some techniques give direct information on material degradation or corrosion rate, while others are used to determine if a corrosive environment may exist. Also, some techniques are "destructive" altering more or less the surface of the metal, while others are nondestructive. The true methods of monitoring the corrosion are considered very sensitive measurements, which give a practical instantaneous signal, simultaneously with the change of the corrosion speed.

To obtain a more complete picture of the corrosion process, it is often necessary to obtain complementary data, from other sources or sensors, which are purchased simultaneously with those obtained from the corrosion sensor.

Three main aspects are pursued in the study of corrosion of alloys in various environments: (1) the type of corrosion involved in the process; (2) the corrosion rate; and (3) the nature of the corrosion products and their properties (chemical, structural, and protective). For this, numerous study methods can be used, which can be divided into three main classes: analytical methods, electrochemical methods, and optical methods. But in special cases, other methods are used (acoustic, nuclear, etc.).

Electrochemical impedance spectroscopy (SIE) data, were processed with the ZSimpWin software [8], in which the spectra are interpreted by the fit procedure developed by Boukamp - by the smallest squares method. In order to process with this software the data acquired by the VoltaMaster 4 program, this were converted by using the EIS file converter program.

The polarization resistance method was used to evaluate the corrosion rate. This method serves to determine the corrosion current, at the corrosion potential of the metal or alloy, from the linear polarization curve obtained for relatively small overvoltages. The corrosion current determined by this method therefore represents the current that appears at the metal/corrosive medium interface when the metal is immersed in the solution and represents the instantaneous corrosion current.

All measurements were made on freshly cleaned surfaces. Each sample was polished on SiC abrasive paper until granulation 2000, degreased with acetone, washed with distilled water, and kept in bidistilled water until introduced into the electrochemical cell.

Figure 11 shows the linear polarization curves in semi-logarithmic coordinates for the samples studied in the Ringer solution, and in **Table 5**, the parameters of instantaneous corrosion in the same physiological environment are presented.

The corrosion potential, E_{cor}, measured in relation to the potential of the saturated calomel electrode, is the potential at which the oxidation-reduction reactions on the surface of the alloy are at equilibrium; the speed of the oxidation reaction is equal to the rate of the reduction reaction, and the total current intensity is zero. As the potential increases toward more positive values, the speed of the oxidation reaction increases, while the movement of the potential toward negative values, the oxidation process is reduced and the metal is passivized. As a qualitative aspect, the TiMoSi alloy series has a higher corrosion tendency than the TiMoZrTa alloys. The differences are significant, and the presence of zirconia and tantalum seems to cause a decrease in the corrosion rate.

The polarization resistors have high values, which are reflected in very low corrosion rates. The product of "corrosion" in the case of these alloys is mainly titanium oxide, TiO_2, which is insoluble and adherent to the surface of the alloy. The oxide layer on the surface protects the alloy from the ages of the electrolytic media. In view of this, it can be admitted that in the artificial physiological environment, Ti-based alloys do not corrode but in fact undergo a passivation process. Under these conditions, the parameter V_{cor}—called corrosion rate—is actually passivation speed.

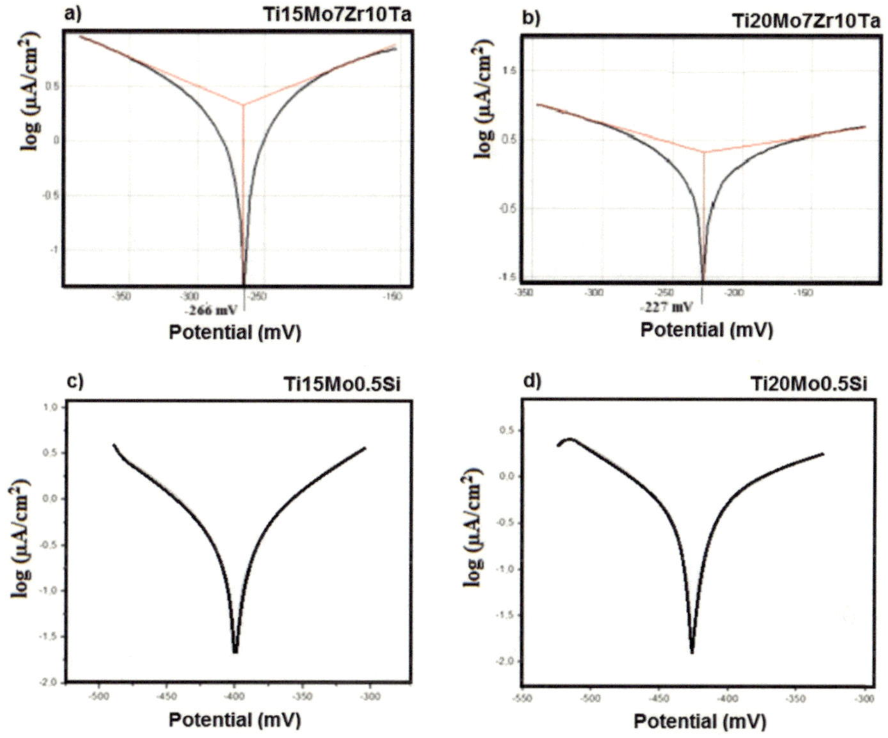

Figure 11.
Linear polarization curves in semi-logarithmic coordinates for titanium alloys developed in Ringer's solution: (a) Ti15Mo0.5Si, (b) Ti20Mo0.5Si, (c) Ti15Mo7Zr10Ta, and (d) Ti20Mo7Zr10Ta.

Alloy element	E_{cor} [mV]	R_p [kΩ/cm²]	J_{cor} [μA/cm²]	V_{cor} [μm /an]	βa [mV]	βc [mV]
Ti15Mo0.5Si	−266	14.91	2.131	20.59	200	−192
Ti20Mo0.5Si	−227	17.71	2.089	20.19	310	−142
Ti15Mo7Zr10Ta	−400.10	46.22	0.37	4.31	92.10	−91.20
Ti20Mo7Zr10Ta	−425.50	50.33	0.38	4.47	130.20	−10.430

Table 5.
Instantaneous corrosion parameters for titanium alloys developed in Ringer's solution.

2.6 Surface characterization

One of the requirements of biomaterials is cellular adhesion on the surface of the material, depending on surface energy. The contact angle between a drop of liquid and a solid surface is a sensitive indicator of changes in surface energy and of the chemical and supramolecular structure on the surface. Specialty studies in domain indicated that contact angle measurement is important for the study of cell adhesion to the surface, being the one that characterizes the hydrophobicity of the studied material [21, 22].

Measurement of the contact angle (**Figure 12**) is an experimental technique used to evaluate the hydrophilic or hydrophobic character of the surfaces. Surfaces can be classified as hydrophilic or hydrophobic reported at 90°. If the angle of contact is between 0 and 90°, the material is hydrophilic, and if the angle of contact is between 90 and 180°, material is hydrophobic.

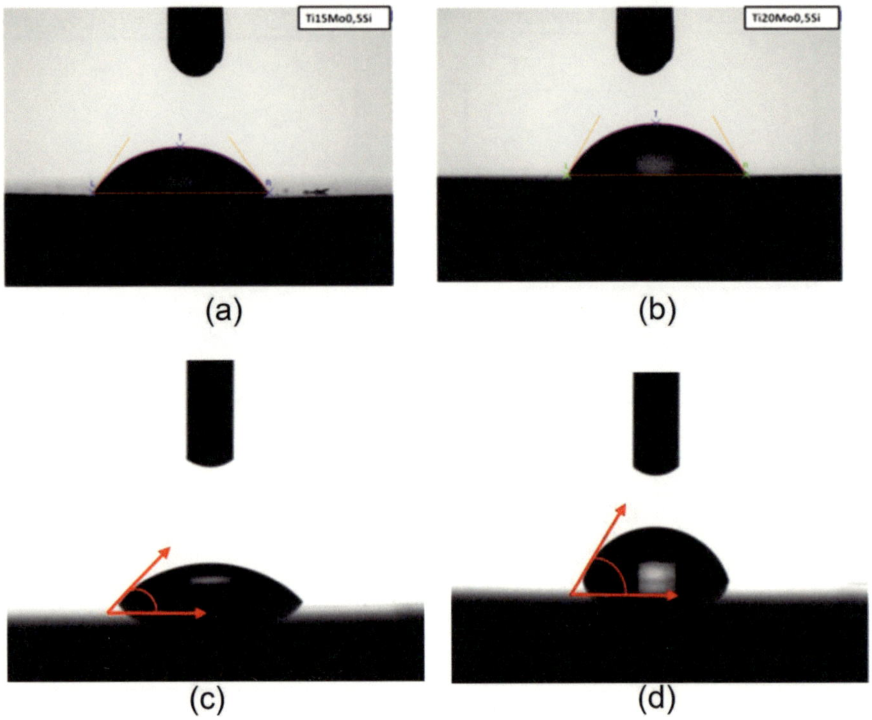

Figure 12.
Images of water droplet on the surface of the elaborated alloys: (a) Ti15Mo0.5Si, (b) Ti20Mo0.5Si, (c) Ti15Mo7Zr10Ta, and (d) Ti20Mo7Zr10Ta.

Alloy	Ti15Mo0.5Si	Ti20Mo0.5Si	Ti15Mo7Zr10Ta	Ti20Mo7Zr10Ta
Liquid used	water	water	water	water
Contact angle (°)	64.40	50.00	45.64	70.72

Table 6.
Water contact angle values on the surface of elaborated titanium alloys.

The equipment used allows the determination of the surface tension of the liquids and of the free surface energy of the solid. The principle of measuring the angle of contact consists in placing a drop of water with a microsurgery syringe with the drop volume of 4 μl. Drop lighting is made from behind and recorded from the opposite side with a digital camera. The image obtained is further analyzed through the FAMAS program, a KYOWA integrated goniometer software.

Ten measurements of the contact angle (θ) for each experimental alloy were performed, and the value presented is the average of the measurements made, with a maximum error of ±1°. The average value of the contact angle for each alloy is shown in **Table 6**.

All investigated alloys have a contact angle of less than 90°, thus having a hydrophilic character, which means a high adhesion of the cells to the surface of the alloys.

From the data obtained for the analyzed titanium alloy surfaces, it follows that the value of the highest arithmetic mean of the alloys is recorded at the level of contact angle with water on the surface of the Ti15Mo7Zr10Ta alloy, and the smallest level was Ti20Mo7Zr10Ta alloy, this alloy having a more pronounced hydrophilic character.

3. Conclusions

Metals have traditionally been used to make implants subjected to high loads in the human body, used in various applications. They are known for their high resistance to wear, ductility, hardness, corrosion, and biocompatibility.

For a biomaterial to be functional for an extended period of time in the body, it should be nontoxic and engage in an adequate response with the body, so that it can fulfill its purpose.

The preliminary investigations presented in this chapter for the elaborated titanium alloys revealed the beneficial influence of some stabilizing β elements (Mo, Ta, and Si).

The alloys developed by the proposed method have the advantage of a modulus of elasticity close to that of the human bone and a good corrosion resistance in the simulated biological fluids. According to the obtained values for corrosion and the mechanical properties, the newly developed alloys, for a Young modulus, the value is the closest to the bone (from 19 to 77 GPa our alloys, C.p. Ti is 105 GPa, and the rest are higher, where the bone is 17 GPa) from all the commercial known alloys, and TMZT systems have the lowest corrosion rate. Also, according to the contact angle, the surfaces of the obtained alloys are susceptible for cell development.

Because improving the properties of biomaterials is a necessity to reduce the failure rate of implants in human tissue, we can say that the alloys developed in this chapter can be successful candidates for orthopedic implants, thanks to the stabilizing β elements.

Author details

Petrică Vizureanu*, Mădălina Simona Bălțatu and Andrei Victor Sandu
Faculty of Materials Science and Engineering, "Gheorghe Asachi" Technical University of Iasi, Iasi, Romania

*Address all correspondence to: peviz2002@yahoo.com

References

[1] Elias CN, Lima JHC, Valiev R, Meyers MA. Biomedical applications of titanium and its alloys. Biological Materials Science. 2008;**60**(3):46-49

[2] Antoniac I, editor. Handbook of Bioceramics and Biocomposites. Springer. 2016. ISBN: 978-3-319-12459-9. Available from: https://www.springer.com/gp/book/9783319124599

[3] Chen Q, Thouas GA. Metallic implant biomaterials. Materials Science and Engineering R. 2015;**87**:1-57

[4] Baltatu MS, Tugui CA, Perju MC, Benchea M, Spataru MC, Sandu AV, et al. Biocompatible titanium alloys used in medical applications. Revista de Chimie. 2019;**70**(4):1302-1306

[5] Geetha M, Singh AK, Asokamani R, Gogia AK. Ti based biomaterials, the ultimate choice for orthopaedic implants—A review. Materials Science. 2009;**54**:397-425

[6] Singh MKK. Review on titanium and titanium based alloys as biomaterials for orthopaedic applications. Materials Science and Engineering: C. 2019;**102**:844-862

[7] Sandu AV, Baltatu MS, Nabialek M, Savin A, Vizureanu P. Characterization and mechanical proprieties of new TiMo alloys used for medical applications. Materials. 2019;**12**(18):2973

[8] Niinomi M. Titanium Alloys. Encyclopedia of Biomedical Engineering. Elsevier. 2019:213-224. DOI: https://doi.org/10.1016/B978-0-12-801238-3.99864-7

[9] Kokubo T, Yamaguchi S. Novel bioactive materials developed by simulated body fluid evaluation: Surface-modifified Ti metal and its alloys. Acta Biomaterialia. 2016;**44**:16-30

[10] Terpiłowska S, Siwicka-Gieroba D, Siwicki AK. Cytotoxicity of Iron (III), Molybdenum (III), and their mixtures in BALB/3T3 and HepG2 cells. Journal of Veterinary Research. 2018;**62**(4):527-533

[11] Correa DRN, Kuroda PAB, Lourenço ML, Fernandes CJC, Buzalaf MAR, Zambuzzi WF, et al. Development of Ti-15Zr-Mo alloys for applying as implantable. Journal of Alloys and Compounds. 2018;**749**:163-171

[12] Bălțatu MS, Vizureanu P, Geantă V, Nejneru C, Țugui CA, Focșăneanu SC. Obtaining and mechanical properties of Ti-Mo-Zr-Ta alloys. IOP Conference Series: Materials Science and Engineering. 2017;**209**(1):012019

[13] Bombac DM, Brojan M, Fajfar P, Kosel F, Turk R. Review of materials in medical applications. Materials and Geoenvironment. 2007;**54**(4):471-499

[14] Shah FA, Thomsen P, Palmquist A. A review of the impact of implant biomaterials on osteocytes. Journal of Dental Research. 2018;**97**(9):977-986

[15] Baltatu MS, Vizureanu P, Balan T, Lohan M, Tugui CA. Preliminary tests for Ti-Mo-Zr-Ta alloys as potential biomaterials, book series. IOP Conference Series: Materials Science and Engineering. 2018;**374**:012023

[16] Niinomi M. Mechanical properties of biomedical titanium alloys. Materials Science and Engineering A. 1998;**243**:231-236

[17] Minciună MG, Vizureanu P, Geantă V, Voiculescu I, Sandu AV, Achiței DC, et al. Effect of Si on the mechanical properties of biomedical CoCrMo alloys. Revista de Chimie. 2015;**66**(6):891-894

[18] Bălţatu MS, Vizureanu P, Mareci D, Burtan LC, Chiruţă C, Trincă LC. Effect of Ta on the electrochemical behavior of new TiMoZrTa alloys in artificial physiological solution simulating in vitro inflammatory conditions. Materials and Corrosion. 2016;**67**(12):1314-1320

[19] Oliveira NTC, Guastaldi AC. Electrochemical stability and corrosion resistance of Ti–Mo alloys for biomedical applications. Acta Biomaterialia. 2009;**5**:399-405

[20] Bălţatu MS, Vizureanu P, Cimpoeşu R, Abdullah MMAB, Sandu AV. The corrosion behavior of TiMoZrTa alloys used for medical applications. Revista de Chimie. 2016;**67**(10):2100-2102

[21] Vogler EA. Structure and reactivity of water at biomaterial surface. Advances in Colloid and Interface Science. 1998;**74**:69-117

[22] Baier RE. Surface behavior of biomaterials: The theta surface for biocompatibility. Journal of Materials Science. Materials in Medicine. 2006;**17**(11):1057-1062

Chapter 5

Impact of Dopants on the Electrical and Optical Properties of Hydroxyapatite

Kumaravelu Thanigai Arul, Jayapalan Ramana Ramya and Subbaraya Narayana Kalkura

Abstract

This chapter deals with the effect of alternating electrical current on hydroxyapatite [HAp, $Ca_{10}(PO_4)_6(OH)_2$] and doped HAp along with their optical response and the processes involved. The dielectric constant, permittivity and ac conductivity were analyzed to have an insight into the surface charge polarization phenomenon. Further, the magnitude and the polarity of the surface charges, microstructure, and phases also play significant role in the cell proliferation and growth on the implants. Besides, the mechanism behind the electrical properties and the healing of bone fracture are discussed. The influence of various dopants on the optical properties of HAp viz., absorbance, transmission, band gaps and defects energy levels are analyzed along with the photoluminescence and excitation independent emission. In the future outlook, the analysis of effect of doping is summarized and its impact on the next generation biomaterials are elucidated.

Keywords: doped hydroxyapatite, electrical, optical, luminescence

1. Introduction

Hydroxyapatite (HAp) is one of the phases of calcium phosphate having excellent biological properties. Human bone contains 75% of inorganic materials (HAp) and remaining organic contents (predominantly collagen) and water. The HAp is analogous to the inorganic compositions of bone. The drawbacks of HAp to be used as an implant (bone and dental replacement material) are its weak mechanical strength, resorbability and to an extent this could be overcome by doping with metal ions. However, there were no adequate new bone formation between living bone and the implants due to the slow osteoconductivity [1]. Even variations in shape, roughness of the implants did not enhance osteoconduction [2]. Some other routes say tissue engineering, even growth factors [bone morphogenic protein (BMP)] [3] etc., also possess some treatment issues. Further, these parameters could not improve the osteoconduction. So, the application of the electric field on the HAp nanoparticles to induce strongly or weakly oriented dipoles, depending on the polarization of the dopants and band gap of the HAp nanoparticles to improve its biocompatibility. Besides, the dopants modify the ionic and space charge polarizations which vary with the ionic size of the dopants.

Recently, many studies have been reported on the electrical properties of HAp/doped HAp. Das and Pamu suggested that HAp could be a suitable candidate for biosensing and micro-electromechanical system applications [4]. The ferroelectric properties of graphene-doped HAp samples were studied by Hendi and Yakuphanoglu [5]. Iron-doped calcium phosphate demonstrated hyperthermia (42°C) within 4 minutes [6]. Study on various metals ions (iron, manganese, and cobalt ions)-doped HAp revealed an increase in the ac conductivity. Further, the annealed iron-doped HAp revealed ferromagnetism, whereas the manganese and cobalt ions doped samples exhibited super-paramagnetic property [7]. The dielectric properties of the chromium-doped HAp were also studied [8]. Various anions such as nitrate, acetate, chloride, and egg shell precursors have been used to prepare HAp particles and their corresponding dielectric constant were 9.96, 13.22, 9.92, and 10.86 at 5 MHz [9]. Porous HAp was prepared from *Pila globosa* shells which possessed high dielectric constant with low dielectric loss [10]. HAp-barium titanate (BT) composite scaffolds having improved electric, compressive strength, toughness, density, and hardness were developed using cold isostatic pressing and sintering by Tavangar et al. [11]. Bismuth ions (10, 30 and 50 wt%) were substituted in the HAp matrix by the conventional solid-state reaction at 1300°C and their ac conductivity was reduced with an increase in Bi content [12]. Space charge and dipolar polarization were the dominant polarization mechanisms in $Na_{0.5}K_{0.5}NbO_3$ (NKN)-HAp as reported by Verma et al. [13]. La, Ba, Fe, and Zn ions doped HAp synthesized by sol-gel route displayed a space charge polarization at low frequency with negative temperature coefficient of resistance [14]. Different contents (e.g., 0, 1, 3, 6, 19, 12, and 15% [wt.]) of gallium ion-doped HAp by microwave-assisted sol-gel technique, illustrated a higher inhibition of bacteria and fungi. Further, gallium ions influence the dielectric properties of HAp [15]. Dielectric properties of chlorinated ethylene propylene diene monomer/hydroxyapatite nanocomposites were robustly distorted at lower frequencies whereas above 103 Hz, it was frequency independent [16]. Horiuchi et al. reported that the polycrystalline HAp possesses conductive grains and insulating grain boundaries further, interfacial polarization was confirmed to be an electret [17]. In the case of chitosan/HAp composite, the concentration of chitosan plays a predominant role in regulating its hardness, conductivity and dielectric constant [18]. HAp particles were permanently polarized by both electric potential (500 V direct current) and thermal treatment (at 1000°C) leading to the high adsorption of inorganic bioadsorbates compared to the as prepared HAp [19]. Electric field assisted sintering such as spark plasma sintering (SPS) and flash sintering (FS) performed on HAp revealed nanovoids within HA grains. Further, in situ TEM heating produced nanovoids which remained stable up to 900°C and were not present at 1100°C [20]. Using sol-gel route, yttrium and strontium co-substituted nano-hydroxyapatite was prepared with a minor phase of β tricalcium phosphate, however the ac conductivity was enhanced with an increase in frequency [21]. Tungsten-doped hydroxyapatite (W-HAp) nanoparticles were prepared by chemical precipitation followed by thermal treatment (800, 1000 and 1200°C) leading to an enhancement in the mechanical strength, Young's modulus and dielectric constant [22]. The synthesis routes, concentration of doping, and doping characteristics affect the behavior of dielectrics as well as other correlated properties such as mechanical and biocompatibility. In the case of doping of semiconductors, the dielectric properties are robustly influenced due to the presence of holes and electrons. When the electric field is applied, the polarization varied in the matrix owing to the occurrence of both holes and electrons. The physical (pressure), chemical (electronic), and thermal treatment significantly alter the properties of HAp leading to the creation of porous, dense and bonded matrix. When electric field is applied to such systems, the electronic polarization, oxygen vacancies, dipole displacement, and atomic orientation are interrelated which alter the permittivity and ac conductivity of HAp. In the case of polymer/HAp composites, the dielectric behavior is distinct due to the presence of carbon and hydrogen chains and the type of bonding. On annealing, the dielectric response of the composites changes significantly due to the formation of voids and porous structures.

Yamashita et al. reported the chemical effects of the electrically polarized HAp in simulated body fluid [23] and in addition enhanced the *in vitro* bioactivity and *in vivo* osteoconductivity [24, 25]. Similarly, the bioactivity of HAp has been improved by doping of metal ions viz., iron [26, 27], silver [28, 29], magnesium [30, 31], strontium [32, 33], etc., in HAp. Co-dopants like magnesium-silver ions [34], iron-zinc [35], etc., have also been used for augmenting physical and biological properties. Electrical and dielectric properties of HAp are crucial for understanding the dipole polarization and surface charge. Depending on the radius of metal ions, substitution or doping takes place in the matrix of HAp which in turn alters the local dielectric polarization leading to micro and macro polarization. Further, these types of polarization modify the surface charges to either positive or negative. In the case of co/tri doping, the basis of lattice has higher atomic and electronic polarization which alter local bonding of the atoms. When electromagnetic field is applied to the co-doped lattice, the wave dispersion is modified when compared to the pristine dielectric material. The ex situ electromagnetic fields enhance the bone fracture healing and bone mineralization [36]. Bowen et al. reported that an enhancement in the barium titanate incorporation in HAp lattice increases the permittivity and ac conductivity [37]. Nakamura et al. revealed the migration of protons along the columnar structure of HAp under electric field at high temperature [38]. Enhanced bone growth was noticed on the negatively charged surface whereas it was reduced on positively charged surface [39]. Osteogenesis was promoted in the dog's jaw-bones using HA-$BaTiO_3$ composites without any change in phase [40]. Nakamura et al. augmented the osteoconduction of the canine bone owing to the bioactive HAp surface as well as accelerated surface charge by electrical polarization [41]. In the lattice of HAp, the hydroxyl atoms were projected along c-axis and charges are modified on application of the electric field and with an increase in temperature. The projection of hydroxyl groups alters to either abundant negative or positive charge that would aid the cell growth and cell proliferation.

The interaction of light with the HAp nanoparticles is another interesting phenomenon, though an insulating material, the presence of phosphate ions aids the emission of photons of different wavelengths. Addition of metal ions in the lattice of HAp tunes the defect energy levels and alters the chemical potential. The dopants can affect the optical and photoluminescence (PL) of HAp. These properties depend on the absorption, transmission, and band gap as well. Further, these properties favor the use of the HAp nanostructure for bio-imaging and biosensing applications. The doped HAp facilitates the trapping of photons at defect sites or ease transmission which enables them for opto-electronic device applications. Popa and Ciobanu reported the enhanced PL by the cerium ions doped HAp without any structural change [42]. The band gap of erbium-doped HAp was reduced displaying red and green emissions [43]. The various emissions were possible due to the formation of defect energy levels coupled with the HAp energy levels which alters the rate of recombination of electron and hole pairs. Further, the doping concentration varies the active centers of recombination. Feng et al. reported that the Eu^{3+}/Gd^{3+}dual-doped HAp nanorods show enhanced PL with a sustained ibuprofen (IBU) release. Further, the nanorods were injected into mice and demonstrated that these nanorods could be used for *in vivo* imaging [44]. Europium-doped HAp revealed high photoluminescence intensity at 900°C due to the migration of europium from Ca1 to Ca2 site [45]. Fluorescent europium-doped HAp nanowires were prepared by hydrothermal technique and in situ dispersion of them for dental applications [46]. Chang et al.

reported dual emission from nitrogen-doped carbon dots (N-CDs)/HAp:europium, gadolinium composite due to aggregation of N-CDs [47]. The nanostructures either one or zero dimensions significantly affect the electronic motion forming many energy levels due to the quantum confinement effect. Moreover, the optical properties of HAp vary on doping of quantum dots, nanowires, etc. When light is shone on the materials, various local emissions occurred that would be absorbed in the matrix subsequently leading to the partial emission of photons. In the case of cerium-doped HAp, the luminescence quenching occurred between the nearest cerium ions in the matrix as reported by Kolesnikov et al. [48]. Various fluoridated HAp doped with Eu^{3+} ion nanoparticles were prepared by hydrothermal technique and the fluorine ions could influence the crystal field environment for luminescence conversion [49]. Reddy et al. observed a strong green emission from Ni^{2+}-doped Ca-Li HAp (CLHA) [50]. Erbium-ytterbium-molybdenum tri-doped HA/β-TCP phosphor was synthesized using solid-state reaction by Van et al. They demonstrated 650 times higher green emission in the presence of molybdenum [51]. In the case of tri-doped HAp, each dopant generates its energy levels and active centers for recombination leading to different emissions. Further, the emission depends on the dopant concentration as well. The praseodymium-doped fluorapatite illustrated green emission at 545 nm and orange emission at 600 nm [52]. Europium/barium co-doped and F-substituted nHAp (HA@nFAp:Eu/Ba) showed high sensitivity in both computed tomography and fluorescence imaging [53]. Carbon dots/HAp/PVA (CDs/HA/PVA) dual-network (DN) hydrogel scaffold showed an excellent fluorescence in non-invasive monitoring field for the in vivo evaluation [54]. In vivo investigation is a challenging task; these advanced materials help in monitoring the cell viability and cell proliferation on implants without following supplementary way to understand cell interaction. Xing et al. developed heparin-coated Eu^{3+}-doped HAp nanoparticles (SH-Eu:nHAP) for bioimaging [55]. HAp nanorods tune color from blue to red and also emit white colors depending on the temperature, excitation wavelengths, etc. [56]. Optical responses, band gap, and emission behavior of materials vary on thermal treatments; further, thermal defects and production of active centers were responsible for the rapid/slow recombination of the electron and hole pairs. Hence, thermal-based luminescence is a fascinating process of emission with respect to various temperatures. However, thermally induced defects are not stable and returned to the ground state by emitting photons. Further, doping modifies the interatomic and intra-atomic transition states of basis during thermoluminescence. For instance, thermoluminescence of HAp doped with different percentages of lanthanum (La), Eu, gadolinium (Gd), and dysprosium (Dy) has been examined under the gamma radiation and (1 m%) Dy-doped samples demonstrated its capability to be used for gamma radiation dosimetry [57]. Cathodoluminescence and thermoluminescence nature of calcium phosphates were also investigated in the UV-IR range with the wavebands due to hydroxyl groups, nonbridging oxygen, etc. [58]. HAp and YAG:Ce ceramics were synthesized by Huang et al. at 850°C to fabricate white light-emitting diodes with phosphor in ceramics (PiCs) color converters in transmission mode [59]. So, these green diodes are useful in reducing the consumption of toxic materials (europium, cadmium etc.) and will guide researchers to develop various green-based diodes. Gd-dependent blue emission was observed on selenium (Se) and gadolinium (Gd) dual ions doped HAp nanoparticles under ultraviolet (UV) irradiation [60]. Copper-doped Sr-HAp was prepared by solid-state reaction $Sr_{10}(VO_4)_{6-x}(PO_4)_xO_2Cu_yH_{2-y-\delta}$ (x = 0–6; y = 0–0.24) as the x value decreases; copper-doped samples show intense blue emission [61]. In most of the cases, the PL emission was reduced due to the concentration quenching and non-radiative recombination of electron and hole pairs which evidently showed the variation of active centers in the matrix.

Europium-doped calcium phosphate apatite-based colloids possess narrow emission with long luminescence lifetimes suitable for nanoprobe as reported by Kattan et al. [62]. These colloids were stable over time and excite near visible or visible light domains. The excited states in the colloids were highly stable and electron decay time was slow. Further, non-radiative recombination centers might be far away from each other to reduce the bleaching effect. Mesoporous strontium ions doped HAp samples exhibited blue emission and sustained drug release [63]. The PL intensity of doped HAp was correlated to the amount of ibuprofen released [63]. Similarly, Yang et al. reported the red emission of europium-doped HAp and its PL intensity altered with the release of drug molecules [64]. This idea has many practical difficulties at *in vivo* level and could be addressed by developing advanced analysis. Thus, doped HAp nanostructures can be an ideal candidate for both bio-imaging and drug delivery. Still, there is a lack of fundamental and basic understanding of electrical and optical nature of doped HAp. The main focus of this chapter is to discuss few instances of metal ions doped HAp and its electrical and optical behavior. Further, the path that lead to the development of next generation advanced biomedical materials will also be examined.

2. Types of calcium phosphates

Calcium phosphates are found in the bone and teeth as the major inorganic constituent. Depending on the Ca/P ratio and structure, the phases of calcium phosphate are classified as tabulated in **Table 1**. Although these phases of calcium phosphate are different from each other by their chemical composition, but they are biocompatible, non-toxic, and osteoconductive in nature which have ability to stimulate tissue regeneration. The HAp and tricalcium phosphate (TCP) are the mostly used ceramics in biomedical applications among the phases of calcium phosphate. The combination of these two phases result in a new phase formation which was recognized as a biphasic calcium phosphate used in bone repair and replacement applications. The phases of calcium phosphate have their individual adsorption and resorption capacities.

S. No.	Phase	Abbreviation	Empirical formula	Ca/P ratio
1.	Calcium phosphate monohydrate	MCPM	$Ca(H_2PO_4)_2.H_2O$	0.5
2.	Monocalcium phosphate	MCP	$Ca(H_2PO_4)_2$	0.5
3.	Dicalcium phosphate	DCP	$CaHPO_4$	1.0
4.	Dicalcium phosphate dihydrate	DCPD	$CaHPO_4.2H_2O$	1.0
5.	Octacalcium phosphate	OCP	$Ca_8H_2(PO_4)_6.5H_2O$	1.33
6.	Tricalcium phosphate	TCP	$Ca_3(PO_4)_2$	1.5
7.	Amorphous calcium phosphate	ACP	$Ca_{10-x}H_{2x}(PO_4)_6(OH)_2$	1.2–2.2
8.	Calcium-deficient hydroxyapatite	CDHA	$Ca_9(HPO_4)(PO_4)_5(OH)$	1.5–1.67
9.	Hydroxyapatite	HAp	$Ca_{10}(PO_4)_6(OH)_2$	1.67
10.	Oxyapatite	OXA	$Ca_{10}(PO_4)_6O$	1.67
11.	Tetracalcium phosphate	TTCP	$Ca_4O(PO_4)_2$	2.0

Table 1.
Phases of calcium phosphate [65].

The solubility of calcium phosphate (CaPs) varies from each other and the *in vivo* degradation was foreseen in the order MCPM>TTCP>α-TCP > DCPD>DCP > OCP > β-TCP > CDHA>HAp [29]. Monocalcium phosphate monohydrate (MCPM) is soluble in water and is acidic in nature. Therefore, it cannot be used in the bone repair applications. The MCPM combined with α-TCP or β-TCP, makes it less soluble [65, 66]. Usually the MCPM has been used as fertilizer and commonly known as superphosphate fertilizer. The Monocalcium phosphate (MCP) was prepared by heating the MCPM at 100–110°C and is similar to the MCPM. The MCP has been rarely used due to its highly hygroscopic nature [67].

Dicalcium phosphate (DCP) is biocompatible and bioresorbable and has been used as bone cement [68, 69]. Dicalcium phosphate dihydrate (DCPD) also known as brushite can be easily synthesized and has osteoconductive property. It is a metastable material and can be converted to other phases DCP, OCP, CDHA, and TCP by varying the pH of the reactant solutions. The octacalcium phosphate (OCP) is responsible for the formation of teeth and bone. It crystallizes very slowly and is not suitable for bone cement application. The α-TCP and β-TCP are polymorphs having same chemical composition with different structures [70, 71]. The α-TCP's solubility is better than that of β-TCP but both are biocompatible, resorbable, and have been used as bone cement. Among the phases of CaPs, the HAp is more stable and highly crystalline in nature. When the HAp is heated above 900°C, it is converted to oxyapatite (OXA) in an inert atmosphere. The tetracalcium phosphate (TTCP) was prepared by heating the DCP and calcium carbonate at 1400°C with rapid cooling [72].

3. Electrical properties

HAp is a bioceramic having a high dielectric constant. Researchers have studied the impact of electric field on the HAp to understand the real part and imaginary part of the permittivity [37, 38]. These properties provide us an insight into the dielectric polarization of electric dipoles with respect to electric field. Further, the dielectric studies aid to understand *in vitro* electrical polarization. The respective real and imaginary part of permittivity grants dispersion of dipoles and energy dissipation. Some other parameters say temperature, experimental condition and dopants can influence and alter the dielectric properties. Doping sites and dopant's radius alter the electronic and orientation polarization, whereas co or tri-doping significantly affects the structure and phase, further, the dielectric properties of these materials might vary due to the rate of dipole relaxation. Generally, at low frequency alternating field, the dielectric constant is high and varies with increase in frequency. Nakamura et al. studied the polarization of HAp using direct current and showed that proton migrates along the columnar OH channel [38]. The polarized charge was high enough to improve biological activity. Usage of the electrical fields enabled the accelerated fracture healing in bones; however, it was slow in the case of long bone [72–74]. There are some reports on electrical stimulation which has been used to enhance the bone growth in spinal fusion [75, 76]. Further, it has been employed to treat osteonecrosis as well as osteoarthritis [77]. The dielectric constant of fluids and tissues in the bone and HAp is crucial for healing. The porosity of HAp plays a vital role for the local electrical field strength [78, 79]. Human bones also contain many elements such as magnesium, zinc, and strontium etc., so, the impact of the elements in the bone also play a vital role in the dielectric constant of bone. Further, it as well depends on the elemental size, concentration, and interrelated porosity.

For instance, doping of magnesium ions on HAp enhances the dielectric constant (**Figure 1A**) [30]. At low frequency, the dielectric constant was high due to ionic polarization; however, it was reduced by lagging of dipoles with respect to electric field. At low magnesium ions doping, the dielectric constant was low and almost equal to the dielectric constant of HAp. So, the low level doping did not highly polarize the ions in the direction of electric field and difficult to locate the dopant site position either at calcium site 1 or calcium site 2. As the Mg concentration increases, both the sites might be occupied and at low frequency the dipoles were strongly oriented, whereas it was disturbed at high frequency. Similarly, the cadmium-doped HAp revealed a higher dielectric constant in comparison with pure HAp. However, 40% of cadmium-doped HAp shows a decrease in the dielectric property. At 1 kHz frequency, the dielectric constant of HAp, doped samples 10 at.% Cd, 20 at.% Cd, 25 at.% Cd, 30 at.% Cd, and 40 at.% Cd were 6.75, 7.12, 8.16, 7.13, 7.26, and 6.24 respectively. At 40 at.% Cd, the structural change from hexagonal to monoclinic with varying crystallinity was responsible for the reduction in the dielectric constant [80]. In the case of silver-doped HAp, the dielectric constant was enhanced due to a high dipole polarization [81]. The dopant size varies the phase of HAp leading to amorphous or partial amorphization which completely modifies the local coordination and chemical potential. Horiuchi et al. revealed the two step relaxations of fluorine substituted HAp (F-HAp) [82]. They depicted that one step from 600 to 60 Hz and other 60 to 20 Hz in HAp which were analogous to the F-HAp. At low frequency, the electric dipoles are largely (L) relaxed, whereas at high frequency, the relaxation was small (S). Further, they calculated the activation energy of HAp and F-HAp as 0.63 and 0.62 eV, respectively, for one type of relaxation and it was independent of fluorine substitution. In case of other relaxation, the activation energy was significantly influenced by fluorine substitution due to the change in orientation of hydroxyl groups [82].

In the case of tungsten (W)-doped HAp, the relative permittivity was reduced up to 1 MHz and from 1 to 5 MHz the permittivity was constant [83]. The dielectric constant of W-doped HAp was high at low frequency due to the polarization of electronic, ionic, dipolar, and space charge. As the doping concentration increases, the dielectric constant was enhanced [83]. Thus, the dopants enhance spreading of the electromagnetic fields in the damaged bone sites or fractured area for rapid healing. Similarly, the other metal ions strontium [21], iron [26] etc., have been used as dopants in HAp to enhance dielectric property. A crucial and impressive part is how dielectric constant varies with concentration and with various dopants and the mechanism involved. The co-doping in HAp leads to the creation of many defects and alters the ionic polarization with respect to electric field. For instance, iron and zinc ions were co-doped in HAp at various concentrations (0.01, 0.05,

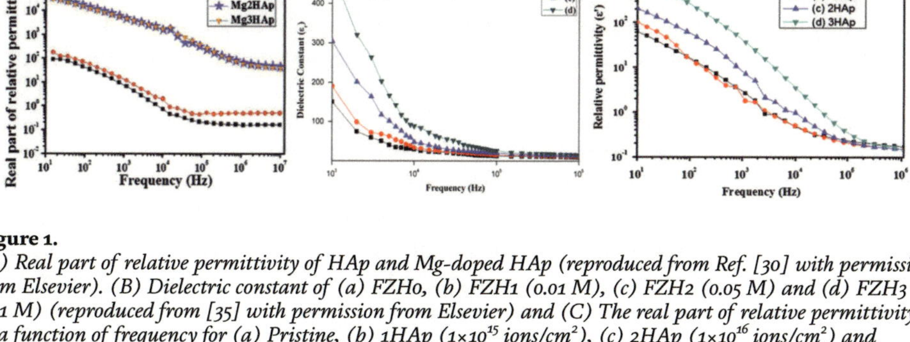

Figure 1.
(A) Real part of relative permittivity of HAp and Mg-doped HAp (reproduced from Ref. [30] with permission from Elsevier). (B) Dielectric constant of (a) FZH0, (b) FZH1 (0.01 M), (c) FZH2 (0.05 M) and (d) FZH3 (0.1 M) (reproduced from [35] with permission from Elsevier) and (C) The real part of relative permittivity as a function of frequency for (a) Pristine, (b) 1HAp (1×10^{15} ions/cm^2), (c) 2HAp (1×10^{16} ions/cm^2) and (d) 3HAp (1×10^{17} ions/cm^2) (reproduced from [84] with permission from Elsevier).

and 0.1 M) by ultrasonication. At higher concentration (FZH3) (0.1M), dielectric constant was greater (**Figure 1B**) compared to the other samples owing to the enhanced ionic polarization and strong orientation of dipoles at low frequency. As the frequency increases, the dielectric constant was reduced in all the samples due to lagging of the dipoles [35]. Generally, at low frequency, the value of dielectric is high due to slow relaxation of dipoles with high orientation. At high frequency, the dielectric constant was reduced due to strong re-alignment of dipoles with field [30, 83]. Further, it depends on the size of dopants, crystal structure, and concentration providing atomic site variations which enable the variations in the unit cell and crystal structure. Moreover, the dopants provide vacancies which affect space charge localization/delocalization. This facilitates the alterations in the dielectric constant. In case of the HAp structure, the hydroxyl ions aligned along c-axis parallel to calcium and phosphate$(PO_4)^{3-}$ ions favor high polarization of electric dipoles thereby increasing the ionic conduction [38]. Surface charge of HAp is another important parameter which assists the bone cell growth. The polarized surface of HAp had improved the osteobonding in canine bone tissues [39]. So, the electric properties have been employed to understand the cellular behavior on bone and to develop bone prostheses [38]. The surface charge of HAp depends on the porosity and dielectric strength. It can vary on low energy ion implantation which are capable of altering the surface properties without affecting the bulk properties of the materials. Nitrogen ions (N^{+1}) were implanted in HAp matrix with varying ion fluences 1×10^{15} (1HAp), 1×10^{16} (2HAp), and 1×10^{17} (3HAp) ions/cm^2 [84]. At higher ion fluence (3HAp), relative permittivity was significantly enhanced (**Figure 1C**) in comparison with other samples because of the higher ionic and space charge polarizations. The surface and subsurface of HAp were modulated on ion implantation altering the dipole polarization thereby leading to the variation in the surface charge of the samples. The polarization varies locally leading to dielectric strength modification at the surface, subsurface and at macro level. Hence, the surface charge can be tuned by different dopants, temperature, and frequency.

The variation of dielectric constant with frequency of pure and Fe-doped HAp, Mn-doped HAp, and Co-doped HAP sample at room temperature was examined by Panneerselvam et.al. [7]. The dielectric constant of the doped samples decreased sharply up to 10 kHz, and then reduced gradually with further increase in frequency. This difference in dielectric constant is due to the four types of polarization such as electronic polarization (frequencies up to 10^{16} Hz), ionic polarization (10^{13} Hz), orientation polarization (up to 10^{10} Hz), and space charge polarization or interfacial (up to 10^3 Hz) [7]. In all the samples, as the doping concentration increases, the dielectric constant was enhanced due to ionic polarization. The highest dielectric constant was exhibited by 5% MnHAp and the lowest by 5% CoHAp [7]. The dopants such as Fe, Mn, and Co possess different ionic radii and electronic cloud density. The variation of dielectric constant of the different metal ions doped HAp is due to the change in dipole strength, rate of dipole relaxation, and space charge polarization apart from ionic polarization. Tavangar et al. fabricated HAp-barium titanate (BT) scaffolds by cold isostatic pressing and sintering. As the BT concentration increases, the dielectric loss (D) of the composite was reduced due to the low porosities and higher densities of composite when compared with pure HAp. The 60 wt% BT had the lowest dielectric loss at 1 kHz. The dielectric constant of the 60 wt% BT–40 wt% HA composite was 46.50 which was the highest compared to the other composites due to the coupling of low-dielectric constant of HA with BT leading to a parallel polarization in the presence of phases with different weight percentages and electrical conductivity [11]. The ac frequency facilitated the coupling of the phases of materials leading to a synergic effect on the dipole polarization and orientation. Verma et al. studied the effect of concentration of piezoelectric $Na_{0.5}K_{0.5}NbO_3$ (NKN) on dielectric and electrical properties of HAp in the range of temperature (30–500°C) at frequency 1 Hz to 1 MHz. The composite was prepared by solid state ceramic method and sintered at 1075°C for 2 h [13]. The experimental values of the dielectric constant are lower than those of calculated using theoretical models [13] due to the connectivity between HAp and NKN phases at the lower concentration of NKN in HAp matrix. The connectivity of matrix and secondary phase affects the electrical as well as mechanical properties of the composites. At low content of NKN, the HAp phases were connected in three-dimension whereas, no connectivity between NKN phases and 0–3 connectivity between NKN and HAp phases were observed. With enhancing content of NKN in the HAp matrix, the interaction between piezoelectric phases was increased. The calculated dielectric values of HAp-10 NKN, HAp-20 NKN, and HAp-30 NKN were 30.54, 38.71 and 50.29 respectively. The effective dielectric constant of HAp-10 NKN, HAp-20 NKN and HAp-30 NKN at 10 kHz (room temperature) were calculated to be 29.81, 35.32 and 42.046 respectively. The calculated and experimental values were significantly varied at high concentrations due to the combined involvement of complex parameters such as orientation and electronic The microstructure, densification, undetectable phases etc. play a vital role in determining the efficient dielectric constant of the composite system [13].

The ac conductivity measurements are used to study the mechanism of hopping and it is a complex phenomenon. Further, it depends on frequency and temperature [30]. The ac conductivity of Mg-doped HAp was enhanced compared to HAp (**Figure 2A**). There was low ac conductivity at low frequency due to the weak turnaround of ions with the electric field. However, it was increased at higher frequency on Mg-doped samples due to the complex array of ions and proton segregation along c-axis [30, 85]. Similar trend also noticed in W-doped HAp samples which linearly depend on the frequency range. Further, it obeyed the universal frequency power law. Towards understanding the mechanism of ac conductivity of the samples, the proverbial Jonscher equation ($\sigma_{ac} = \sigma_{dc} + B\omega^s$) was used [86], where B-constant, ω-angular frequency and s-frequency exponent. Using the slope of lnσ vs. lnω_{ac} and the s values were calculated as 1.0622, 1.0600, 1.0623, 1.0501, 1.0518, 1.0629, and 1.0534 for pure and 1, 5, 10, 20, 30, and 40% of W in HAp, respectively. Here, s is almost ≤1, revealing no measureable direct current conductivity and displays prompt hopping with a translational motion [83]. In the case of the Cd-doped HAp samples, the alternating current conductivity was enhanced from 10^{-10} to 10^{-5} s cm^{-1} with an increase in frequency. The frequency exponent(s) was

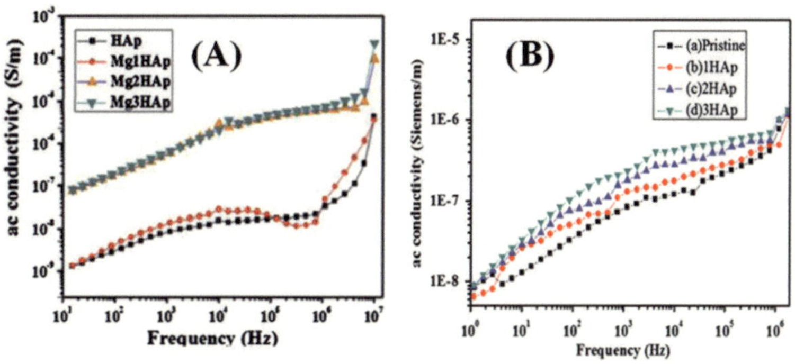

Figure 2.
(A) Ac conductivity as a function of frequency of HAp and Mg-doped HAp (reproduced from Ref. [30] with permission from Elsevier); and (B) The ac conductivity as a function of frequency for (a) Pristine, (b) 1HAp, (c) 2HAp and (d) 3HAp (reproduced from [84] with permission from Elsevier).

determined from the slope of logσ vs. logω and its value equal to 1 for the samples [80]. Eventually, it displays a lack of direct current conductivity [87]. Similar, s value was realized for the Te-doped HAp samples however, their ac conductivity enhanced at low concentration due to $s \geq 1$ leading to localized hopping. At higher concentration, it was reduced due to $s \leq 1$ leading to translation motion with a rapid hopping motion [88]. Ion implantation could also be employed to alter the ac conductivity, without using expensive and toxic chemicals. It can precisely modulate the ac conductivity up to a particular depth. Nitrogen ions implanted samples demonstrated higher ac conductivity at higher frequency owing to the strong arrangement of complex ions compared to pristine (**Figure 2B**). However, it was less at low frequency due to the weak turnover of ions [84].

4. Optical properties

The interaction of light on materials leads to transmission, absorptions and reflection. These parameters depend on refractive index, wavelength, dielectric constant, and dopants. Dopants play a vital role in creating the abundant defects/vacancies in the lattice of materials. When light interacts on the bound charges of the materials, they either transmit or reflect back. The structure and phase of HAp varied depending on the type of dopant [80] which also alters the optical properties of HAp. The optical properties of HAp were enhanced by developing smaller grains and low porosity in the HAp matrix. It is an optically anisotropic material and possesses a refractive index in the range 1.644 and 1.651 depending on light polarization and direction of propagation [89]. A highly transparent HAp nanosized grains were used to observe *in vivo* interactions with proteins/cells [90, 91]. For a proper insight of the optical properties, intrinsic correlated parameters/quantities say crystalline structure, dispersion of phonon, band structure, dielectric response, band gap, etc. are required. Density functional theory displays a local or semi local exchange-correlation interaction of HAp providing a band gap between 4.5 and 5.4 eV depending on the type of valence states [92, 93]. However, the (semi) local exchange-correlation underestimates the band gap of HAp, and thus its value is above 5.5 eV [94]. So, the defect free HAp is transparent to visible light under middle or far ultraviolet illumination having a band gap >6 eV. Interesting point to note is that the dopants produce defects level in between conduction band and valence band.

For instance, the thenoyltrifluoroacetonate (TTA)- and europium (Eu)-doped HAp were used to enhance transmission spectra by 20% compared to PMMA. The TTA shows a red shift and the transmission edge from 275 to 375 nm. Both the TTA and HAp mixture restrict the formation of PMMA clusters improving the transparency. In this case, the absorption and scattering losses were introduced by the TTA and the HAp nanoparticles [95]. The other example, Cd-doped HAp showed enhanced reflectivity at the Cd (40 at.%) due to the structural transformation to the monoclinic phase. Further, it alters the refractive index of the samples as well [80]. At a particular atomic percentage, the structural transformation occurred affecting the electronic polarization thereby, altering the reflectivity. In the case of erbium doping in HAp, seven absorption bands were noticed [43]. The bands observed at 1520, 980, 803, 657, 524, 490, and 448 nm corresponding to the electronic transitions from ground state $^4I_{15/2} \rightarrow {}^4I_{13/2}$, $^4I_{15/2} \rightarrow {}^4I_{11/2}$, $^4I_{15/2} \rightarrow {}^4I_{9/2}$, $^4I_{15/2} \rightarrow {}^4F_{9/2}$, $^4I_{15/2} \rightarrow {}^2H_{11/2}$, $^4I_{15/2} \rightarrow {}^4F_{7/2}$, and $^4I_{15/2} \rightarrow {}^4F_{3/2}$, respectively [92]. Among all the transitions, the $^4I_{15/2} \rightarrow {}^2H_{11/2}$ transition had the highest intensity due to the hypersensitive transition [92]. Further, the peaks were broadened inhomogeneously due to the f-f

DOI: http://dx.doi.org/10.5772/intechopen.93092

interactions of Er^{3+} ions [96]. As the erbium doping concentration increases, the intensity of the peaks increased due to the replacement of Ca^{2+} by Er^{3+} ions. Further, there was a blue shift observed on the doped HAp due to the reduced particle size [97]. The Er-HAp samples possess direct band gap (n = 1/2) so band to band transitions was allowed. As the erbium doping concentration increased, the band gap was enhanced to 4.46 eV from 4.02 eV. Hence the structure, phase, defects and particle size of HAp are the key parameters to alter either the absorption or reflection. Further, the symmetry of the HAp also plays a predominant role in modifying the electronic polarization and dielectric constant.

Apurba et al. studied the optical response of HAp films of various thicknesses on amorphous SiO_2 substrates [98]. All the films showed 75–96% transparency in the visible region. There are two regions noticed, one is absorption and other a transparent oscillating region. Below 300 nm, the transmittance of the HAp films displayed robust absorption. When the film thickness enhances, the absorption edge was shifted to higher wavelength in turn altering electronic polarization Thus, these films revealed a strong absorption in UV region and transparency in the visible regions as well. The band gap of the varying thickness of HAp thin films was in the range 5.25–4.67 eV due to an increase in crystallinity and grain size. The band gap of thin films is similar to the band gap of bulk HAp (in the range of 5.4 to 4.51) [99]. For annealed films, the refractive indices were augmented with an increase in the film thickness [98]. Flores et al. reported that using the Kubelka-Munk function through the maximum of the first derivative, the absorption edge values were 5.62, 4.74 and 4.6 eV which correspond respectively to TbW0 [calcium-deficient (CD) HAp], TbW10 (terbium 10%-doped CDHA), and TbW12 (terbium 20%-doped CDHA) [100]. The optical band gap values of the TbW0, TbW10 and TbW12 samples were 5.41, 4.49 and 4.38 eV respectively. This demonstrates that as the Tb increases, the band gap was reduced. Here the host matrix having calcium vacancies was considered as n-type, whereas the Tb acts as a p-type dopant. When the Tb ions substitute at that calcium site then the electrons were delocalized to conduction band. Further, in the case of the TbW10 and TbW12 samples, the band gap was reduced. From the UV photoelectron spectra, the valence band energies of Ev0 (TbW0), Ev1 (TbW10) and Ev2 (TbW12) were 3.33, 2.55 and 2.40 eV, respectively [100]. It exhibits a decrease in the valence band at the higher concentration of Tb and varies Fermi level of the samples.

Feng et al. studied the drug adsorption capacity of HAp using absorption spectra [44, 101]. The respective drug adsorption capacity of the undoped HAp nanorod and the Eu^{3+}/Gd^{3+} HAp was 653.5 and 841.4 mg/g. The interaction of the dopants with drug molecules might be strong due to the presence of oxygen vacancies and atomic defects which pave a path for sustained or rapid release of drug molecules. This revealed that the doped nanorods displayed a high drug adsorption compared to undoped sample with a reduced absorbance. The size of the dopant and its doping concentration play a predominant role in modifying the crystal structure thereby the Fermi level position gets altered leading to the enhancement or decrease of the band gap. When photon interacts with the material, either high absorbance or transmission of photons occurs due to the variation in energy levels of defects or vacancies. The optical response of the doped HAp is not only dependent on material property and type of dopant (drug or organic molecules) but also on the type of wavelength used. Moreover, different wavelengths have distinct capability of light reflection, absorbance, and transmission as well.

The carbon-based HAp showed enhanced optical absorption. N-doped carbon dots (N-CDs) revealed absorption at about 240 and 340 nm, due to the Π–Π* transition of C = C and Π–Π* transition of C = O and C–N/C = N, respectively [56].

In the case of HAp:Eu,Gd, the absorption at 200–280 nm due to the wide band gap of HAp with a peak (395 nm), was assigned to the intrinsic 4f-4f transition absorption of Eu [56] confirming the incorporation of Eu into HAp. The absorption of N-CDs/HAp:Eu,Gd was superior than single N-CDs and HAp:Eu,Gd and its band edge shifted to 550 nm due to the porous structure and multiple reflection [47]. The CDs based system could be used as a stable bioimaging candidate. Ni^{2+}-doped calcium-lithium hydroxyapatite (CLHA) nanopowders were synthesized by mechanochemical synthesis by Reddy et al. [50]. The spectra of these powder possess four absorption band at 420, 718, 794, and 1189 nm attributed to the transitions of $^3A_{2g}(F) \rightarrow {}^3T_{1g}(P)$, $^3T_{1g}(F)$, $^1E_{1g}(D)$ (spin-forbidden transition), and $^3T_{2g}(F)$, respectively [50]. The chemical potential of the CLHA is drastically affected leading to the modification of conductivity and dielectric properties. Iron, manganese, and cobalt ions doped HAp possess direct band gap (index number n = 1/2). The band gap of 5% Co-doped HAp was higher than Fe, Mn ions doped samples [7]. The band gaps were modified due to the presence of defect energy levels which shift Fermi level toward the valence or conduction band.

5. Photoluminescence

The PL of HAp depends on the defect energy level formation, structure, and size of the nanoparticle. Moreover, its band gap is above 5.5 eV, when dopants added to HAp matrix, the band gap perhaps vary due to the formation of many defects energy levels in between valence and conduction band. When the HAp nanostructure was excited by different wavelengths, electrons were accordingly excited to the higher states sometimes, these electrons recombine with holes promptly to produce radiative emission. However, in some cases, the emission might be non-radiative. Proper understanding of the effect of dopant is required to create either light active or inactive centers which enable emission at different wavelengths. However, it also depends on the excitation wavelength as well. The defects energy level formation is a complex phenomenon containing the associated band position and the band bending process. It as well depends on the size, phase and atomic arrangements. In order to reduce non-radiative emission, the doping concentration must be properly tuned to avoid the occurrence of concentration quenching; otherwise, abundant non-radiative centers are facilitated [34].

Addition of sodium hydroxide (NaOH) varies PL of Sr-HAp samples [102]. By varying NaOH content, the shape of the spectra did not change drastically; however, the intensities vary significantly. The Sr-HAp sample (0.15 g NaOH) displays the strongest emission and the weakest intensity was at 0.40 g NaOH due to the variation in luminescent centers. Here, neither Sr^{2+} nor PO_4^{3-} is responsible for the luminescence but it was due to the carbon and oxygen related active electronic defect centers on the host matrix [102]. Some reports are available for the self-activated luminescence due to the addition of trisodium citrate which enables the creation of carbon monoxide impurities [103]. In the case of the Tb-doped samples, the excitation peaks of TbW10 (terbium 10% CDHA) and TbW12 (terbium 20% CDHA) were matched with that of CDHA. Further, the vacancies and carbonate radicals act as acceptor chromophores and terbium ions as donor chromophores. The interaction of chromophores leads to a non-radiative relaxation through defects and impurities in each sample [100]. Two different wavelengths (255 and 264 nm) were used for excitation of the samples. The emission peaks were associated with $^5D_4 \rightarrow {}^7F_6$ (489 nm), $^5D_4 \rightarrow {}^7F_6$ (544 nm), $^5D_4 \rightarrow {}^7F_4$ (585 nm), and $^5D_4 \rightarrow {}^7F_3$ (622 nm) due to intraconfigurational 4f-5d transitions of the Tb^{3+} ion. At the 544 nm, a high intense green light emission was noticed in the doped samples

(TbW10) [104, 105]. There was a weak contribution of the PL emission from the host matrix of both samples and displayed a deformation of the peak shape with a small shift in the peaks $^5D_4 \rightarrow {}^7F_6$ and $^5D_4 \rightarrow {}^7F_4$ transitions. The emission from TbW10 was high due to chemical composition, self-activated CDHA, whereas at higher Tb doping (TbW12), the intensity was reduced due to concentration quenching leading to non-radiative relaxation [100].

Yang et al. reported the broad excitation spectrum at 250 nm due to the charge transfer between europium and oxygen ions and further, small peaks were noticed at longer wavelength due to f-f transitions of Eu^{3+} [28]. It was monitored by $^5D_0 \rightarrow {}^7F_2$ transition at 612 nm. The two peaks were prominently noticed at $^5D_0 \rightarrow {}^7F_1$ (590 nm) and $^5D_0 \rightarrow {}^7F_2$ (612 nm). Even the IBU-loaded europium-doped HAp samples display a clear PL spectrum and it can be tracked by the luminescence intensity. The fascinating part is how the PL intensity varies with release rate of drug molecules. As the cumulative release rate increases, the PL intensity enhances and reached maximum when all drug molecules were released completely. The organic groups of the IBU highly quenched the emission due to europium in the IBU-Eu:HAp. The IBU creates high non-radiative centers in the matrix. However, the release of IBU augments with a weakening of quenching effect which was confirmed by enhanced PL intensity. Thus, it was used as a potential probe for monitoring the drug release [28].

In the case of dual ions doped samples, the europium/gadolinium dual-doped HAp nanorods showed a maximum excitation peak at 394 nm [44]. There was no significant emission on the co-doping of europium (Eu^{3+})/gadolinium (Gd^{3+}) compared to the lone europium doping. However, the PL intensity was altered and four emission peaks were noticed at 590, 615, 650, and 699 nm [44]. The prominent peak was identified at 615 nm due to $^5D_0 \rightarrow {}^7F_2$ transition within Eu^{3+} ions. The other PL peaks were observed at 590, 650, and 699 nm owing to their respective $^5D_0 \rightarrow {}^7F_1$, $^5D_0 \rightarrow {}^7F_3$, and $^5D_0 \rightarrow {}^7F_4$ transitions. As the doping concentration of europium increases, the PL emission intensity was enhanced. The highest PL intensity occurred in 5 mol% Eu^{3+} but with an enhanced intensity compared to the dual doped samples. The PL intensity was higher at the doping ratio of Eu^{3+} to Gd^{3+} (1:2) than the ratio 1:1. On UV irradiation, the dual doped samples displayed a robust red emission from powder as well as from powder dispersed solution [44]. So, the PL intensity depends on the phase, particle size and defect based active centers which absolutely alter either the inter- or intra band transition and emission.

In the case of Mg ions doping on HAp, the PL intensity was enhanced accompanied by a modification of the spectra. At higher Mg concentration, the peak was reduced due to weak radiative recombination [30]. Further, the defects create many active centers for non-radiative recombination and the centers might be very close to each other for a rapid decrease in the PL intensity. As the Mg and Ag ions in HAp augments, the PL intensity was enhanced, however, as the concentration raises, the intensity was reduced (**Figure 3A**) [34]. With further increase in co-doping, the PL intensity was enhanced but lesser than the lowest concentration of co-doping [34]. A similar emission was also seen in the iron and zinc co-incorporated HAp samples, but as the co-doping increases, the PL intensity was reduced (**Figure 3B**) [35]. So, the PL intensities were tuned by varying co-doping concentration which might alter the radiative recombination active center in the HAp matrix. Ion implantation is one of the effective routes to dope a particular element at the desired depth and varying defects energy level to tune the PL intensity. Nitrogen ion implantation enhanced the PL emission of HAp [84]. As the ion fluence increases, the PL intensity was enhanced due to the radiative recombination of electron-hole pair without the influence of concentration quenching effect (**Figure 3C**) [84]. There are reports on different synthesis routes for doping of various elements on HAp viz., microwave-assisted

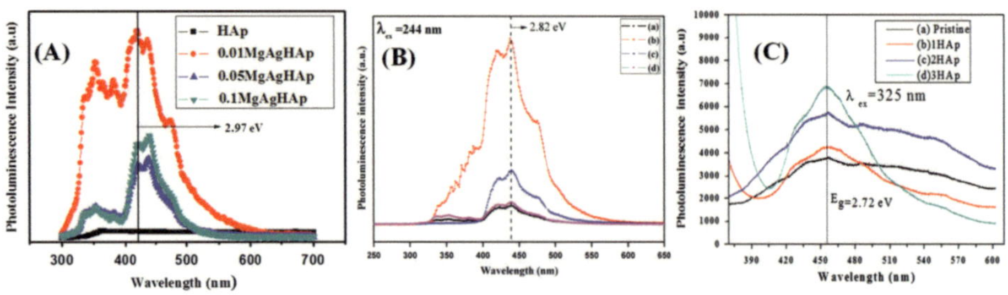

Figure 3.
(A) Photoluminescence spectra of HAp and magnesium and silver ions co-incorporated HAp samples (reproduced from [34] with permission from Elsevier), (B) Photoluminescence spectra of (a) FZH0, (b) FZH1, (c) FZH2 and (d) FZH3 (reproduced from [35] with permission from Elsevier) and (C) Photoluminescence of (a) pristine, (b) 1HAp, (c) 2HAp and (d) 3HAp (reproduced from [84] with permission from Elsevier).

route followed by ion implantation which is similar to dual ions doping [106]. However, the implantation was used to create/dope ions on the surface and subsurface with associated defects/vacancies without disturbing bulk properties of HAp. For instance, nitrogen ion implantation on magnesium ion incorporated HAp samples demonstrated that at low fluence of nitrogen, the PL intensity was enhanced [106]. However, at high fluence, the intensity was reduced due to concentration quenching and high non-radiative centers created on the surface. The PL intensity of unmodified Mg-doped HAp decreased drastically compared to the surface modified samples [106]. In the case of polymer (polyvinyl alcohol) doping in HAp, the PL intensity was raised [107] and the highest PL intensity was noticed at higher concentration due to the formation of abundant active sites created by the carbon and oxygen radicals in the polymer chains. So, the PL signal could be enhanced by optimizing the doping concentration, varying the band gap and creating active recombination defect sites and vacancies.

Machado et al. studied the photoluminescence of HAp nanorods at different excitation wavelengths (380 to 680 nm) [56]. They demonstrated a shift of emission from blue to red owing to the absence of the short wavelength emission with an increase in the excitation. Near-UV excitation, the intensity was higher with blue/green emissions. Eventually, the best emission intensity was in the range 330 to 430 nm [56]. Erbium-ytterbium (Yb)-molybdenum (Mo) tri-doped HA/β-TCP phosphor prepared by solid-state reaction was examined for intense green upconversion (UC) emission [51]. M5 ((0.5% mol) Er-(10% mol) Yb-(8% mol) Mo tri-doped HA/β-TCP) showed green emission intensity 650 times than that of the M1 (0.5% mol Er-doped HA/β-TCP), M2 ((0.5% mol) Er-(10% mol) Yb co-doped HA/β-TCP) due to energy transfer from $^2F_{7/2}$, $^3T_2$ > state of Yb^{3+} – $MoO_4{}^{2-}$ dimer to the $^4F_{7/2}$ of Er^{3+} ions. Further, red emission was weak because of feeble absorption cross-section of $^4I_{13/2}$ and the green emission band can be controlled by the Mo^{6+} doping concentrations. It aids to use the material for bioimaging application [51]. N-doped carbon dots/HAp:Eu,Gd (N-CDs/HAp:Eu,Gd) composite were studied [47] and the PL spectra of N-CDs/HAp:Eu,Gd simultaneously revealed the emission from N-CDs and HAp:Eu,Gd on single wavelength excitation. The PL emission depicted no shift under different wavelengths revealing excitation independent emission. It clearly shows that the electronic structure of N-CDs and Eu ions were not affected during the synthesis. So, both the N-CDs and HAp:Eu,Gd were preserved. The PL lifetime of both N-CDs/HAp:Eu,Gd and N-CDs illustrated a single exponential decay but the lifetime decreased from 11.7 ns (N-CDs) to 5.6 ns (N-CDs/HAp:Eu,Gd) owing to the photogenerated charges [47]. Further, it could be used for bioimaging with distinct differentiation of colors due to different emission from carbon dots and doped HAp samples. Polymer/inorganic based structures can also affect the PL. Karthikeyan et al.

described the formation of core-shell structures on argon ion implanted polymer-based zinc ions incorporated HAp and reported that the zinc ions and the polymer lead to formation of many defects which in turn produces additional energy states. The PL intensity at the lower fluence samples (1×10^{14} ions/cm^2) showed enhancement in the PL intensity due to the presence of higher radiative active centers. On increasing the fluence viz., 1×10^{15} ions/cm^2 and 1×10^{16} ions/cm^2, the PL intensity was decreased owing to the formation of more non-radiative centers [108]. The incorporation of metal ions such as iron not only play a major role in tailoring the optical properties but also when exposed to magnetic field, they tend to change their morphologies depending on the magnetic field strength and have potential biological application such as protein absorption [109]. It could also lead to the development of magnetic based prolonged PL emission. Hence, the structure and morphology play a prominent role in altering the radiative/non-radiative recombination sites which can be correlated to the PL intensity decay.

6. Summary and future outlook

The effect of electric field, electromagnetic dispersion, dielectric relaxation and correlated structural variation of the doped HAp samples was discussed. The role of hydroxyl ions, frequency exponent and the mechanism of ac conductivity by translation and hopping motion in the doped HAp samples were elaborated. Further, the electrical studies showed that the polarized surface charge either positive or negative, could alter the growth of bone cells on HAp. The surface charge, microstructure, densification, porosity, phase, electrical dipole reversal and its strong orientation were responsible for the enhancement in the dielectric constant of the doped HAp samples. The optical response depends on the dopant size and its concentration and associated phase transformation. The formation of different energy levels and electronic level transitions on doping enabled the tuning of the PL intensity and multi-color emissions which are independent of the excitation wavelength. The drug-loaded doped HAp samples and their PL intensity were correlated to the rate of drug release. Thus, the europium ion-doped HAp behaves as a one-dimensional nanoprobe for tracking the drug release. Further, different synthesis routes, doping, and co-doping are capable of generating new energy levels between conduction and valence band. Moreover, it was understood that the respective radiative and non-radiative emission were due to the activated luminescent centers and the concentration quenching of the doped samples.

Electro-opto biomaterials could be developed for the rapid healing of bone defects and fracture owing to the enhanced bone cell proliferation and growth. Current, *in vitro* and *in vivo* analysis routes must be improved further to control infection and to enhance the cell growth after implantation. To have an exact biomimicking of the bone, multielemental incorporation of the HAp is essential. Still, there is a lack of advanced analysis technique to have an insight of the surface charge interaction with the bone cells and how these charges assist the precipitation, mineralization, and growth of bone tissues. Solar/photon and magneto/light-based advanced biomaterials need to be developed for rapid healing and recovery.

Acknowledgements

The authors thank AMSS, IGCAR, Kalpakkam, Tamil Nadu, for providing the lab facilities to carry out the characterization of the samples.

Author details

Kumaravelu Thanigai Arul[1*], Jayapalan Ramana Ramya[2] and
Subbaraya Narayana Kalkura[3*]

1 Energy and Biophotonics Laboratory, Department of Physics, AMET (Deemed to be University), Chennai, Tamil Nadu, India

2 National Centre for Nanoscience and Nanotechnology, University of Madras, Guindy Campus, Chennai, Tamil Nadu, India

3 Crystal Growth Centre, Anna University, Chennai, Tamil Nadu, India

*Address all correspondence to: thanigaiarul.k@gmail.com and kalkura@yahoo.com

References

[1] Soballe K, Larsen ST, Gelineck J, Fruensgaard S, Hansen ES, Ryd L, et al. Migration of hydroxyapatite coated femoral prostheses. Journal of Bone and Joint Surgery. 1993;**75-B**:681-687

[2] Chang YL, Stanford CM, Wefel JS, Keller JC. Osteoblastic cell attachment to hydroxyapatite-coated implant surfaces in vitro. The International Journal of Oral & Maxillofacial Implants. 1999;**14**:239-247

[3] Schilephake H. Bone growth factors in maxillofacial skeletal reconstruction. International Journal of Oral and Maxillofacial Surgery. 2002;**31**:469-484

[4] Das A, Pamu D. A comprehensive review on electrical properties of hydroxyapatite based ceramic composites. Materials Science and Engineering: C. 2019;**101**:539-563

[5] Hendi AA, Yakuphanoglu F. Dielectric and ferroelectric properties of the graphene doped hydroxyapatite ceramics. Journal of Molecular Structure. 2020;**1207**:127734

[6] Baskar S, Elayaraja K, Nivethaa EAK, Ramya JR, Sankar VD, Catalani LH, et al. Thermally modified iron-inserted calcium phosphate for magnetic hyperthermia in an acceptable alternating magnetic field. Physical Chemistry B. 2019;**123**:5506-5513

[7] Panneerselvam R, Anandhan N, Gopu G, Roselin AA, Ganesan KP, Marimuthu T. Impact of different transition metal ions in the structural, mechanical, optical, chemico-physical and biological properties of nanohydroxyapatite. Applied Surface Science. 2020;**506**:144802

[8] Ibrahim M, Dawood A. Influence of doping chromium ions on the electrical properties of hydroxyapatite. Egyptian Journal of Basic and Applied Sciences (EJBAS). 2020;**7**:35-46

[9] Sundarabharathi L, Ponnamma D, Parangusan H, Chinnaswamy M, Maadeed MAAA. Effect of anions on the structural, morphological and dielectric properties of hydrothermally synthesized hydroxyapatite nanoparticles. SN Applied Sciences. 2020;**2**:94

[10] Nayak B, Misra PK. Recognition of the surface characteristics and electrical properties of a nanocrystalline hydroxyapatite synthesized from *Pila globosa* shells for versatile applications. Materials Chemistry and Physics. 2019;**230**:187-196

[11] Tavangar M, Heidari F, Hayati R, Tabatabaei F, Vashaee D, Tayebi L. Manufacturing and characterization of mechanical, biological and dielectric properties of hydroxyapatite-barium titanate nanocomposite scaffolds. Ceramics International. 2020;**46**:9086-9095

[12] Khouri AE, Zegzouti A, Elaatmani M, Capitelli F. Bismuth-substituted hydroxyapatite ceramics synthesis: Morphological, structural, vibrational and dielectric properties. Inorganic Chemistry Communications. 2019;**110**:107568

[13] Verma AS, Kumar D, Dubey AK. Dielectric and electrical response of hydroxyapatite – $Na_{0.5}K_{0.5}NbO_3$ bioceramic composite. Ceramics International. 2019;**45**:3297-3305

[14] Helen S, Kumar AR. Study of structural, mechanical and dielectrical properties of ions doped apatite for antibacterial activity. Materials Chemistry and Physics. 2019;**237**:121867

[15] Obaid A, Omer K, Mai HSA, Zahran HY, Kilany M, Yahia IS, et al. Antimicrobial activity of Ga-doped hydroxyapatite nanostructures: Synthesis, morphological,

spectroscopic, and dielectric properties. Journal of Biomaterials and Tissue Engineering. 2019;**9**:881-889

[16] Nihmath A, Ramesan MT. Preparation, characterization, thermal, and electrical properties of chlorinated ethylene propylene diene monomer/ hydroxyapatite nanocomposites. Polymer Composites. 2016;**39**:1-8

[17] Horiuchi N, Madokoro K, Nozaki K, Nakamura M, Katayama K, Nagai A, et al. Electrical conductivity of polycrystalline hydroxyapatite and its application to electret formation. Solid State Ionics. 2018;**315**:19-25

[18] Sanchez AG, Prokhorov E, Barcenas GL, García AGM, Y, Muñoz EMR, Raucci MG, Buonocore G. Chitosan-hydroxyapatite nanocomposites: Effect of interfacial layer on mechanical and dielectric properties. Materials Chemistry and Physics. 2018;**217**:151-159

[19] Rivas M, Valle LJD, Armelin E, Bertran O, Turon P, Puiggalí J, et al. Hydroxyapatite with permanent electrical polarization: Preparation, characterization, and response against inorganic adsorbates. ChemPhysChem. 2018;**19**:1746-1755

[20] Yun J, Qin W, Benthem KV, Thron AM, Kim S, Han YH. Nanovoids in dense hydroxyapatite ceramics after electric field assisted sintering. Advances in Applied Ceramics. 2018;**117**:376-382

[21] Lakshmanaperumal S, Mahendran C. Structural, dielectric, cytocompatibility, and in vitro bioactivity studies of yttrium and strontium co-substituted nano-hydroxyapatite by sol–gel method. Journal of Sol-Gel Science and Technology. 2018;**88**:296-308

[22] Maiti M, Sarkar D, Liu S, Xu S, Maiti B, Paul K, et al. Tungsten doped hydroxyapatite processed at different temperatures: Dielectric behaviour and anti-microbial properties. New Journal of Chemistry. 2018;**42**:16948-16959

[23] Yamashita K, Oikawa N, Kitagaki K, Umegaki T. Acceleration and deceleration of bone-like crystal growth on ceramic hydroxyapatite by electrical poling. Chemistry of Materials. 1996;**8**:12697-12700

[24] Ueshima M, Tanaka S, Nakamura S, Yamashita K. Manipulation of bacterial adhesion and proliferation by surface charges of electrically polarized hydroxyapatite. Journal of Biomedical Materials Research. 2002;**60**:578-584

[25] Ohgaki M, Kizuki T, Katsura M, Yamashita K. Manipulation of selective cell adhesion and growth by surface charges of electrically polarized hydroxyapatite. Journal of Biomedical Materials Research. 2001;**57**:366-373

[26] Mercado DF, Magnacca G, Malandrino M, Rubert A, Montoneri E, Celi L, et al. Paramagnetic iron-doped hydroxyapatite nanoparticles with improved metal sorption properties. A bioorganic substrates-mediated synthesis. ACS Applied Materials & Interfaces. 2014;**6**:3937-3946

[27] Silvia P, Monica M, Monica S, Michele I, Alessio A, Martina G, et al. Magnetic labelling of mesenchymal stem cells with iron-doped hydroxyapatite nanoparticles as tool for cell therapy. Journal of Biomedical Nanotechnology. 2016;**12**:909-921

[28] Stanica V, Janackovic D, Dimitrijević S, Tanasković SB, Mitrić M, Pavlović MS, et al. Synthesis of antimicrobial monophase silver-doped hydroxyapatite nanopowders for bone tissue engineering. Applied Surface Science. 2011;**257**:4510-4518

[29] Trujillo NA, Oldinski RA, Ma H, Bryers JD, Williams JD, Popat KC.

Antibacterial effects of silver-doped hydroxyapatite thin films sputter deposited on titanium. Materials Science and Engineering: C. 2012;**32**:2135-2144

[30] Arul KT, Elayaraja K, Manikandan E, Bhalerao GM, Chandra VS, Ramya JR, et al. Green synthesis of magnesium ion incorporated nanocrystalline hydroxyapatite and their mechanical, dielectric and photoluminescence properties. Materials Research Bulletin. 2015;**67**:55-62

[31] Ziani S, Meski S, Khireddine H. Characterization of magnesium-doped hydroxyapatite prepared by sol-gel process. International Journal of Applied Ceramic Technology. 2014;**11**:83-91

[32] Nan K, Wu T, Chen J, Jiang S, Huang Y, Pei G. Strontium doped hydroxyapatite film formed by micro-arc oxidation. Materials Science and Engineering: C. 2009;**29**:1554-1558

[33] Avci M, Yilmaz B, Tezcaner A, Evis Z. Strontium doped hydroxyapatite biomimetic coatings on Ti6Al4V plates. Ceramics International. 2017;**43**:9431-9436

[34] Arul KT, Ramya JR, Bhalerao GM, Kalkura SN. Physicochemical characterization of the superhydrophilic, magnesium and silver ions co-incorporated nanocrystalline hydroxyapatite, synthesized by microwave processing. Ceramics International. 2014;**40**:13771-13779

[35] Ramya JR, Arul KT, Elayaraja K, Kalkura SN. Physicochemical and biological properties of iron and zinc ions co-doped nanocrystalline hydroxyapatite, synthesized by ultrasonication. Ceramics International. 2014;**40**:16707-16717

[36] Hoepfner TP, Case ED. The porosity dependence of the dielectric constant for sintered hydroxyapatite. Journal of Biomedical Materials Research. 2002;**60**:643-650

[37] Bowen CR, Gittings J, Turner IG, Baxter F, Chaudhuri JB. Dielectric and piezoelectric properties of hydroxyapatite-$BaTiO_3$ composites. Applied Physics Letters. 2006;**89**:132906

[38] Nakamura S, Takeda H, Kimihiro U. Proton transport polarization and depolarization of hydroxyapatite ceramics. Journal of Applied Physics. 2001;**89**:5386

[39] Kobayashi T, Nakamura S, Yamashita K. Enhanced osteobonding by negative surface charges of electrically polarized hydroxyapatite. Journal of Biomedical Materials Research. 2001;**57**:477-484

[40] Feng JQ, Yuan HP, Zhang XD. Promotion of osteogenesis by a piezoelectric biological ceramic. Biomaterials. 1997;**18**:1531-1534

[41] Nakamura S, Kobayashi T, Yamashita K. Extended bioactivity in the proximity of hydroxyapatite ceramic surfaces induced by polarization charges. ournal of Biomedical Materials Research. 2002;**61**:593-599

[42] Popa CL, Ciobanu CS. Synthesis and characterization of fluorescent hydroxyapatite. Romanian Reports in Physics. 2016;**68**:1170-1177

[43] Ammar ZA, Muhammed A, Goh YF, Rafiq M, Kadir A, Abdolahi A, et al. Structural characterization, optical properties and in vitro bioactivity of mesoporous erbium-doped hydroxyapatite. Journal of Alloys and Compounds. 2015;**645**:478-486

[44] Feng C, Peng H, Zhu YJ, Wu J, Zhang CL, Cui DX. The photoluminescence, drug delivery and imaging properties of multifunctional Eu^{3+}/Gd^{3+} dual-doped

hydroxyapatite nanorods. Biomaterials. 2011;**32**:9031-9039

[45] Baldassarre F, Altomare A, Corriero N, Mesto E, Lacalamita M, Bruno G, et al. Crystal chemistry and luminescence properties of Eu-doped polycrystalline hydroxyapatite synthesized by chemical precipitation at room temperature. Crystals. 2020;**10**:250

[46] Li L, Li D, Zhao W, Cai Q, Li G, Yu Y, et al. Composite resin reinforced with fluorescent europium-doped hydroxyapatite nanowires for in-situ characterization. Dental Materials. 2020;**36**:e15-e26

[47] Chang Q, Xu W, Chen Q, Xue C, Li N, Yang J, et al. One step synthesis of N-doped carbon dots/hydroxyapatite:EuGd composite with dual-emissive and solid-state photoluminescence. Applied Surface Science. 2020;**508**:144862

[48] Kolesnikov IE, Nikolaev AM, Lähderanta E, Frank-Kamenetskaya OV, Kuz'mina MA. Structural and luminescence properties of Ce^{3+}-doped hydroxyapatite nanocrystalline powders. Optical Materials. 2020;**99**:109550

[49] Zhang X, Xing Q, Liao L, Han Y. Effect of the fluorine substitution for –OH group on the luminescence property of Eu^{3+} doped hydroxyapatite. Crystals. 2020;**10**:191

[50] Reddy CV, Ravindranadh K, Ravikumar RVSSN, Shim J. A novel green-emitting Ni^{2+}-doped Ca-Li hydroxyapatite nanopowders: Structural, optical, and photoluminescence properties. Journal of Materials Science: Materials in Electronics. 2020;**31**:5097-5106

[51] Van HN, Vu NH, Pham VH, Huan PV, Hoan BH, Nguyen DH, et al. A novel upconversion emission material based on Er^{3+}–Yb^{3+}–Mo^{6+} tridoped hydroxyapatite/tricalcium phosphate (HA/β-TCP). Journal of Alloys and Compounds. 2020;**827**:154288

[52] Milojkov DV, Silvestre OF, Vojislav Dj S, Janjić GV, Mutavdžić DR, Milanović M, et al. Fabrication and characterization of luminescent Pr^{3+} doped fluorapatite nanocrystals as bioimaging contrast agents. Journal of Luminescence. 2020;**217**:116757

[53] Zhou R, Li Y, Xiao D, Li T, Zhang T, Fub W, et al. Hyaluronan-directed fabrication of co-doped hydroxyapatite as a dual-modal probe for tumor-specific bioimaging. Journal of Materials Chemistry B. 2020;**8**:2107-2114

[54] Wang Y, Xue Y, Wang J, Zhu Y, Wang X, Zhang X, et al. Biocompatible and photoluminescent carbon dots/hydroxyapatite/PVA dual-network composite hydrogel scaffold and their properties. Journal of Polymer Research. 2019;**26**:248

[55] Xing Q, Zhang X, Wu D, Han Y, Wickramaratne MN, Dai H, et al. Ultrasound-assisted synthesis and characterization of heparin-coated Eu^{3+} doped hydroxyapatite luminescent nanoparticles. Journal of Colloid and Interface Science. 2019;**29**:17-25

[56] Machado TR, Leite IS, Inada NM, Li MS, da Silva JS, Andres J, et al. Designing biocompatible and multicolor fluorescent hydroxyapatite nanoparticles for cell-imaging applications. Materials Today Chemistry. 2020;**14**:100211

[57] Daneshvar H, Shafaei M, Manouchehri F, Kakaei S, Ziaie F. The role of La, Eu, Gd, and Dy lanthanides on thermoluminescence characteristics of nano-hydroxyapatite induced by gamma radiation. SN Applied Sciences. 2019;**1**:1146

[58] Barrera-Villatoro A, Boronat C, Rivera-Montalvo T, Correcher V,

Garcia-Guinea J, Zarate-Medina J. Cathodo- and thermally stimulated luminescence characterization of synthetic calcium phosphates. Spectroscopy Letters. 2018;**51**:22-26

[59] Huang P, Zhou B, Zheng Q, Tian Y, Wang M, Wang L, et al. Nano wave plates structuring and index matching in transparent hydroxyapatite-YAG:Ce composite ceramics for high luminous efficiency white light-emitting diodes. Advanced Materials. 2020;**32**:1905951

[60] Luo H, Xie J, Xiong L, Yang Z, Zuo G, Wang H, et al. Engineering photoluminescent and magnetic lamellar hydroxyapatite by facile one-step Se/Gd dual-doping. Journal of Materials Chemistry B. 2018;**6**:3515

[61] Pogosova MA, González LV. Influence of anion substitution on the crystal structure and color properties of copper-doped strontium hydroxyapatite. Ceramics International. 2018;**44**:20140-20147

[62] Al-Kattan A, Pascal D, Jeannette DG, Christophe D. Preparation and physicochemical characteristics of luminescent apatite-based colloids. Journal of Physical Chemistry C. 2010;**114**:2918-2924

[63] Zhang C, Li C, Huang S, Hou Z, Cheng Z, Yang P, et al. Self-activated luminescent and mesoporous strontium hydroxyapatite nanorods for drug delivery. Biomaterials. 2010;**31**:3374-3383

[64] Yang P, Quan Z, Li C, Kang X, Lian H, Lin J. Bioactive, luminescent and mesoporous europium-doped hydroxyapatite as a drug carrier. Biomaterials. 2008;**28**:4341-4347

[65] Bohner M. Calcium orthophosphates in medicine: From ceramics to calcium phosphate cements. Injury. 2000;**31**:37-47

[66] Constantz BR, Ison IC, Fulmer MT, Poser RD, Smith ST, Wagoner MV, et al. Skeletal repair by in situ formation of the mineral phase of bone. Science. 1995;**267**:1796-1799

[67] Benard J. Combinaisons avec le phosphore. In: Benard E, Bouissieres G, Brusset H, et al., editors. Nouveau trait6 de chimieminerale. Vol. 4. Paris: Masson; 1958. pp. 455-488

[68] Costantino PD, Friedman CD, Jones K, Chow LC, Pelzer HJ, Sisson GA Sr. Hydroxyapatite cement. I. Basic chemistry and histologic properties. Archives of Otolaryngology – Head & Neck Surgery. 1991;**117**:379-384

[69] Friedman CD, Costantino PD, Jones K, Chow LC, Pelzer HJ, Sisson GA. Hydroxyapatite cement. II. Obliteration and reconstruction of the cat frontal sinus. Archives of Otolaryngology – Head & Neck Surgery. 1991;**117**:385-389

[70] Khairoun I, Driessens FC, Boltong MG, Planell JA, Wenz R. Addition of cohesion promotors to calcium phosphate cements. Biomaterials. 1999;**20**:393-398

[71] Ciesla K, Rudnicki R. Synthesis and transformation of tetracalcium phosphate in solid state. Part I. Synthesis of roentgenographically pure tetracalcium phosphate from calcium dibasic phosphate and calcite. Polish Journal of Chemistry. 1987;**61**:719-727

[72] Kaygili O, Dorozhkin SV, Ates T, Ghamdi AA, Yakuphanoglu F. Dielectric properties of Fe doped hydroxyapatite prepared by sol–gel method. Ceramics International. 2014;**40**:9395-9402

[73] Ryaby JT. Clinical effects of electromagnetic and electric fields on fracture healing. Clinical Orthopaedics. 1998;**355**:S205-S215

[74] Scott G, King JB. A prospective, double-blind trial of electrical

capacitive coupling in the treatment of nonunion of long bones. The Journal of Bone and Joint Surgery. American Volume. 1994;**76A**:820-826

[75] Oishi M, Onesti ST. Electrical bone graft stimulation for spinal fusion: A review. Neurosurgery. 2000;**47**:1041-1055

[76] Goodwin CB, Brighton CT, Guyer RD, Johnson JR, Light KI, Yuan HA. A double-blind study of capacitively coupled electrical stimulation as an adjunct to lumbar spinal fusions. Spine (Phila Pa 1976). 1999;**24**:1349-1357

[77] Otter MW, McLeod KJ, Rubin CT. Effects of electromagnetic fields in experimental fracture repair. Clinical Orthopaedics and Related Research. 1998;**355**:S90-S104

[78] Marino AA, Becker RO, Bachman CH. Dielectric determination of bound water of bone. Physics in Medicine and Biology. 1967;**12**:367-378

[79] Lakes RS, Harper RA, Katz JL. Dielectric relaxation in cortical bone. Journal of Applied Physics. 1977;**48**:808-811

[80] Kaygili O, Keser S, Ates T, Ghamdi AA, Yakuphanoglu F. Controlling of dielectrical and optical properties of hydroxyapatite based bioceramics by Cd content. Powder Technology. 2013;**245**:1-6

[81] Iqbal N, Kadir MRA, Malek NANN, Mahmood NHB, Murali MR, Kamarul T. Characterization and antibacterial properties of stable silver substituted hydroxyapatite nanoparticles synthesized through surfactant assisted microwave process. Materials Research. 2013;**48**:3172-3177

[82] Horiuchi N, Endo J, Nozaki K, Nakamura M, Nagai A, Katayama K, et al. Dielectric evaluation of fluorine substituted hydroxyapatite. Journal of the Ceramic Society of Japan. 2013;**121**:770-774

[83] Shkir M, Kilany M, YahiaI S. Facile microwave-assisted synthesis of tungsten-doped hydroxyapatite nanorods: A systematic structural, morphological, dielectric, radiation and microbial activity studies. Ceramics International. 2017;**43**:14923-14931

[84] Thanigairul K, Elayaraja K, Magudapathy P, Mudali UK, Nair KGM, Sudarshan M, et al. Surface modification of nanocrystalline calcium phosphate bioceramic by low energy nitrogen ion implantation. Ceramics International. 2013;**39**:3027-3034

[85] ShKalil M, Beheri HH, Fattah WIA. Structural and electrical properties of zirconia/hydroxyapatite porous composites. Ceramics International. 2002;**28**:451-458

[86] Jonscher AK. The 'universal' dielectric response. Nature. 1977;**267**:673-679

[87] Dyre JC, Schrøder TB. Universality of ac conduction in disordered solids. Reviews of Modern Physics. 2000;**72**:873-892

[88] Yahia IS, Shkir M, AlFaify S, Ganesh V, Zahran HY, Kilany M. Facile microwave-assisted synthesis of Te-doped hydroxyapatite nanorods and nanosheets and their characterizations for bone cement applications. Materials Science and Engineering C. 2017;**72**:472-480

[89] Holzmann D, Holzinger D, Hesser G, Schmidt T, Knor G. Hydroxyapatite nanoparticles as novel low-refractive index additives for the long-term UV-photoprotection of transparent composite materials. Journal of Materials Chemistry. 2009;**19**:8102-8106

[90] Kotobuki N, Ioku K, Kawagoe D, Fujimori H, Goto S, Ohgushi H. Observation of osteogenic differentiation cascade of living mesenchymal stem cells on transparent hydroxyapatite ceramics. Biomaterials. 2005;**26**:779-785

[91] Eriksson M, Liu Y, Hu J, Gao L, Nygren M, Shen Z. Transparent hydroxyapatite ceramics with nanograin structure prepared by high pressure spark plasma sintering at the minimized sintering temperature. Journal of the European Ceramic Society. 2011;**31**:1533-1540

[92] Calderin L, Stott M, Rubio A. Electronic and crystallographic structure of apatites. Physical Review B. 2003;**67**:134106

[93] Rulis P, Ouyang L, Ching WY. Electronic structure and bonding in calcium apatite crystals: Hydroxyapatite, fluorapatite, chlorapatite, and bromapatite. Physical Review B. 2004;**70**:155104

[94] Slepko A, Demkov AA. First-principles study of the biomineral hydroxyapatite. Physical Review B. 2011;**84**:134108

[95] Wiglusz RJ, Bednarkiewicz A, Strek W. Synthesis and optical properties of Eu^{3+} ion doped nanocrystalline hydroxyapatites embedded in PMMA matrix. Journal of Rare Earths. 2011;**29**:1111-1116

[96] Mahraz ZAS, Sahar MR, Ghoshal SK, Dousti MR. Concentration dependent luminescence quenching of Er^{3+}-doped zinc boro-tellurite glass. Journal of Luminescence. 2013;**144**:139-145

[97] Pan A, Yang Z, Zheng H, Liu F, Zhu Y, Su X, et al. Changeable position of SPR peak of Ag nanoparticles embedded in mesoporous SiO_2 glass by annealing treatment. Applied Surface Science. 2003;**205**:323-328

[98] Apurba D, Kumar AC, Bharti GP, Behera RR, Mamilla RS, Khare A, et al. Effect of thickness on optical and microwave dielectric properties of hydroxyapatite films deposited by RF magnetron sputtering. Journal of Alloys and Compounds. 2018;**739**:729-736

[99] Matsunaga K, Kuwabara A. First-principles study of vacancy formation in hydroxyapatite. Physical Review B. 2007;**75**:014102

[100] Flores YJ, Quezada MS, Trigos JBR, Rojas LL, Suarez V, Mantilla A. Characterization of Tb-doped hydroxyapatite for biomedical applications: Optical properties and energy band gap determination. Journal of Materials Science. 2017;**52**:9990-10000

[101] Ma MY, Zhu YJ, Li L, Cao SW. Nanostructured porous hollow ellipsoidal capsules of hydroxyapatite and calcium silicate: Preparation and application in drug delivery. Journal of Materials Chemistry. 2008;**18**:2722-2727

[102] Zhanglei N, Zhidong C, Wenjun LI, Changyan S, Jinghua Z, Yang L. Solvothermal synthesis and optical performance of one-dimensional strontium hydroxyapatite nanorod. Chinese Journal of Chemical Engineering. 2012;**20**:89-94

[103] Zhang CM, Yang J, Quan ZW, Yang PP, Li CX, Hou ZY, et al. Hydroxyapatite nano- and microcrystals with multiform morphologies: Controllable synthesis and luminescence properties. Crystal Growth & Design. 2009;**9**:2725-2733

[104] Ling L, Yukan L, Jinhui T, Ming Z, Haihua P, Xu X, et al. Surface modification of hydroxyapatite nanocrystallite by a small amount of terbium provides a biocompatible fluorescent probe. Journal of Physical Chemistry C. 2008;**112**:1229-12224

[105] Han Y, Wang X, Li S, Ma X. Synthesis of terbium doped calcium phosphate nanocrystalline powders by citric acid sol–gel combustion method. Journal of Sol-Gel Science and Technology. 2009;**49**:125-129

[106] Arul KT, Ramya JR, Vanithakumari SC, Magudapathy P, Mudali UK, Nair KGM, et al. Novel ultraviolet emitting low energy nitrogen ion implanted magnesium ion incorporated nanocrystalline calcium phosphate. Materials Letters. 2015;**153**:182-185

[107] Arul KT, Ramya JR, Karthikeyan KR, Kalkura SN. A novel and rapid route to synthesize polyvinylalcohol/calcium phosphate nanocomposite coatings by microwave assisted deposition. Materials Letters. 2014;**135**:191-194

[108] Karthikeyan KR, Arul KT, Ramya JR, Nabhiraj PY, Menon R, Krishna JBM, et al. Core/shell structures on argon ions implanted polymer based zinc ions incorporated HAp nanocomposite coatings. Materials Science in Semiconductor Processing. 2019;**104**:104687

[109] Baskar S, Ramya JR, Arul KT, Nivethaa EAK, Mahadevan Pillai VP, Kalkura SN. Impact of magnetic field on the mineralization of iron doped calcium phosphates. Materials Chemistry and Physics 2018;**218**:166-171

Chapter 6

Biomaterial for Bone and Dental Implants: Synthesis of B-Type Carbonated Hydroxyapatite from Biogenic Source

Bernard Owusu Asimeng, David Walter Afeke and Elvis Kwason Tiburu

Abstract

There are several sources from which hydroxyapatite (HAp) can be obtained and may be broadly categorized as synthetic or biogenic. Elevated interest in recent times has pushed for the development of several procedures for extracting HAp from biogenic wastes due to their excellent composition and morphology resemblance to the human calcified tissue (B-type carbonated HAp). Notable biogenic sources reported for HAp extraction span bovine bones, fish scales, corals, egg-shells, and snails among other calcium-rich sources. However, most of the synthetic methods are laborious and therefore result in high production costs. In this chapter, we discuss the synthesis of B-type carbonate substituted HAp from an untapped biogenic source, *Achatina achatina* shells, using a simple precipitation method and a controlled heat-treatment method. This unique treatment method affected the substitution resulting in different crystallographic parameters and revealed a novel material for bone implants and enamel applications.

Keywords: biogenic source, biomaterial, carbonated hydroxyapatite

1. Introduction

Hydroxyapatite (HAp) is a member of the calcium apatite (group of phosphate) family with a high concentration of hydroxyl group [1–3]. Stoichiometric HAp, $Ca_{10}(PO_4)_6(OH)_2$ can exhibit either monoclinic or hexagonal crystal structures [4, 5]. The most frequently reported hydroxyapatite crystal structure is the hexagonal system, which consists of unconnected, PO_4^{3-} tetrahedra with Ca^{2+} in the interstitial space and a chain of OH^- ions along the c-axis to balance the unit cell charges [4]. This hexagonal crystal structure allows for replacement (substitution) of ions into the structure. The substitution makes the HAp more reactive and biocompatible [6, 7]. The human calcified tissue (e.g., bone and tooth enamel) consists of mineral components similar to carbonated HAp (CHAp) [8, 9]. As a result, extensive research has been conducted to substitute carbonate into commercial HAp to achieve a suitable material for hard tissue replacement and implants coatings [10, 11].

There are two main types of carbonate (CO_3) substitution that occur in hydroxyapatite, namely A-type and B-type. A-type occurs when CO_3 replaces OH groups, while B-type substitution occurs when CO_3 replaces PO_4 in the apatite structure. If these substitutions take place concurrently, an AB-type substitution occurs. Among the types of substitution, literature reports that B-type CHAp is highly similar to the human calcified tissue, which contains 3–5 wt% of carbonate in the lattice of the phosphate [12–15].

Laboratories have advanced in methods for the synthesis of B-type CHAp but the methods are laborious and expensive. For example, the method most frequently reported in the literature is the one proposed by LeGeros [16]. Herein, the preparation begins by adding PO_4/CO_3 solution in a stepwise manner into $Ca(NO_3)_2{\cdot}4H_2O$ solution at a temperature of 90°C. The mixture is stirred for 5 h at a pH of 11 and the precipitates filtered and dried for 10 h at 100°C in an oven. The B-type CHAp is then identified using X-ray diffractometry (XRD) and infra-red (IR) spectrometry. The XRD is a good analytical tool to study the substitution since; CO_3 has a smaller planar ion diameter than the tetrahedral PO_4 group, and thus the substitution of CO_3 with PO_4 will result in a decrease of the a-axis and a small increase in the c-axis of the unit cell. On the other hand, in a narrow range, vibrating bonds of functional groups in a material vibrate with a characteristic wavenumber [17], which is why IR spectroscopy is used to study the functional groups.

In this chapter, the authors discussed a simple precipitation and heat treatment method for the preparation of B-type CHAp from *Achatina achatina* (AA) shells and phosphate-containing solution. Additionally, the XRD and IR results obtained for the substitution are discussed.

2. Obtaining calcite from the AA shells for HAp preparation

Achatina achatina (AA) is the giant African snail ubiquitously scattered throughout the African continent particularly in West Africa, Ghana. The land strata of the soil are made up of various ions, and the eating habit of the snails enables the ingestion of these ions into their shells in trace amounts. The AA shells, however, serve as a rich source of calcium carbonate ($CaCO_3$)—a precursor for HAp preparation compared to other biogenic sources like bovine bones, fish scales, corals, eggshells, and other landmark snail shells. $CaCO_3$ mainly exists in two crystal forms: aragonite and calcite. The aragonite structure as indicated by the XRD pattern in **Figure 1(a)** exists in 'raw ground' AA shells after the shells are washed with running water to remove sludge and dried in the open air for 6 h. The structure contains impurities like sulphate (SO_4^{2-}) and is indicated in the IR spectra in **Figure 2(a)**. These impurities consequently rule out raw AA powders as carbonate precursors for the HAp formation. Thus, the raw AA powder is calcined at high temperatures to burn the impurities and convert the aragonite structure into calcite. The calcination temperature typically used is between 600 and 800°C [18] [see **Figure 1(b)–(d)**]. The IR spectra in **Figure 2(b)** and **(c)** support XRD patterns, which show that the temperatures (600 and 700°C) facilitate the conversion of the aragonite structure to calcite. The calcite functional groups occur at wavenumbers 712, 856, and 1418 cm^{-1}. The calcite structure is formed at the two temperatures, however, the ideal calcination temperature for HAp synthesis is between 800 and 850°C. These temperatures bring an additional phase to the calcite to initiate the HAp preparation. The evidence is shown in **Figure 2(d)** where a dual-phase of calcite and calcium hydroxide [$Ca(OH)_2$] is observed. The calcite absorbed moisture from the atmosphere during the open-air drying; so, under high temperature (800°C) the $CaCO_3$ decomposes to form $Ca(OH)_2$. The reaction pathway is given by **Eqs. (1)** and **(2)**:

$$CaCO_3 + H_2O \xrightarrow{heat(800°C)} CaO.H_2O + CO_2\uparrow \quad (1)$$

$$CaO.H_2O \rightarrow Ca(OH)_2 \tag{2}$$

The reaction is confirmed with IR results in **Figure 2(d)** showing the hydroxyl group (OH^-) of calcium hydroxide at wavenumber 3642 cm^{-1}, and calcium oxide (Ca—O bonding) stretches from wavenumbers 400 to 700 cm^{-1} in calcite.

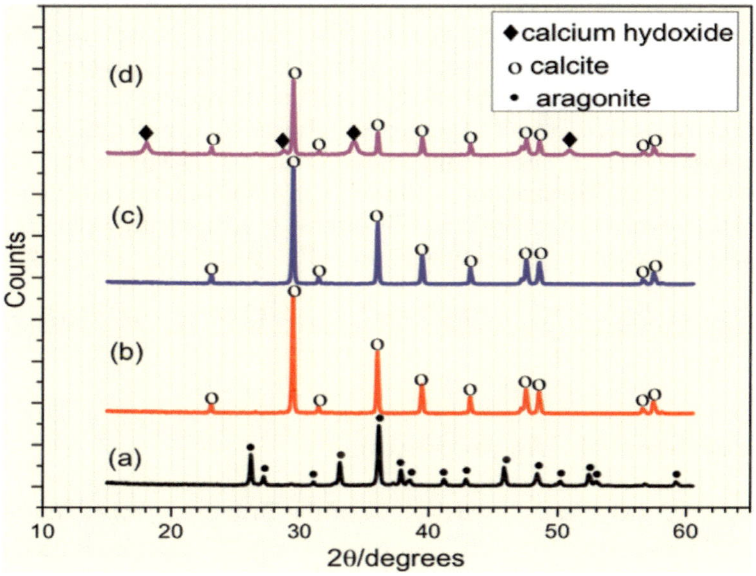

Figure 1.
XRD patterns of (a) raw uncalcined AA powder and (b) calcined AA powder at 600°C (c) 700°C (d) 800°C.

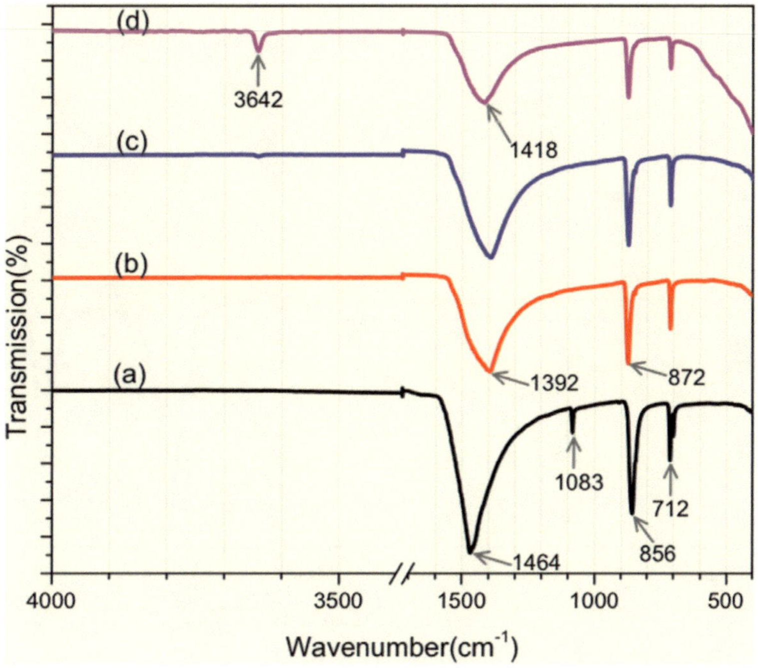

Figure 2.
IR spectra of (a) raw uncalcined AA powder and (b) calcined AA powder at 600°C (c) 700°C and (d) 800°C.

3. HAp preparation

HAp is prepared from 0.3 M solution of diammonium hydrogen phosphate (DHP, pH of 8.12) and 5.7 g of calcite. The calcite is dissolved in distilled water of volume 0.15 cm^3 and the same volume of calcite is measured for DHP. The DHP is then added stepwise while stirring at 40°C for 1 h. The stirring time controls the particle size. The longer the stirring time the smaller the particle size [14]. The calcite mostly preferred for HAp preparation has $Ca(OH)_2$ phase; so, in aqueous solution, the $Ca(OH)_2$ quickly dissociates into $2Ca^{2+}$ and $2OH^-$, whereas $(NH_4)_2HPO_4$ produces $(NH_4)_2OH$ and a monophosphoric acid (HPO_4). The monophosphoric acid reacts with OH groups released by the calcium hydroxide to form a phosphate ester through a condensation reaction. The phosphate ester reacts with Ca to form HAp. The reaction is allowed to age for 24 h to enable HAp crystals growth [14]. The ammonium hydroxide is filtered together with water to obtain the HAp crystals. The reaction pathway is given in Eq. (3):

$$10Ca(OH)_2 + 6(NH_4)_2.HPO_4 + 2H_2O \rightarrow Ca_{10}(PO_4)_6(OH)_2 + 12NH_4OH_{(l)} + 8H_2O \quad (3)$$

4. B-type carbonated HAp preparation

The calcite ($CaCO_3$) in the mixed-phase of the HAp precursor decomposes into calcium (Ca^{2+}) and carbonate (CO_3^{2-}) during stirring. The calcium is used as part of the HAp formation and the CO_3^{2-} lies behind the lattice of phosphate (PO_4^{3-}). The ionic diameter of PO_4^{3-} is larger than that of CO_3^{2-}, thus the first masked the latter and is not detected using XRD. The IR spectra in **Figure 3(a)** show major functional groups of HAp and minor functional groups of carbonate. The PO_4^{3-} groups of HAp

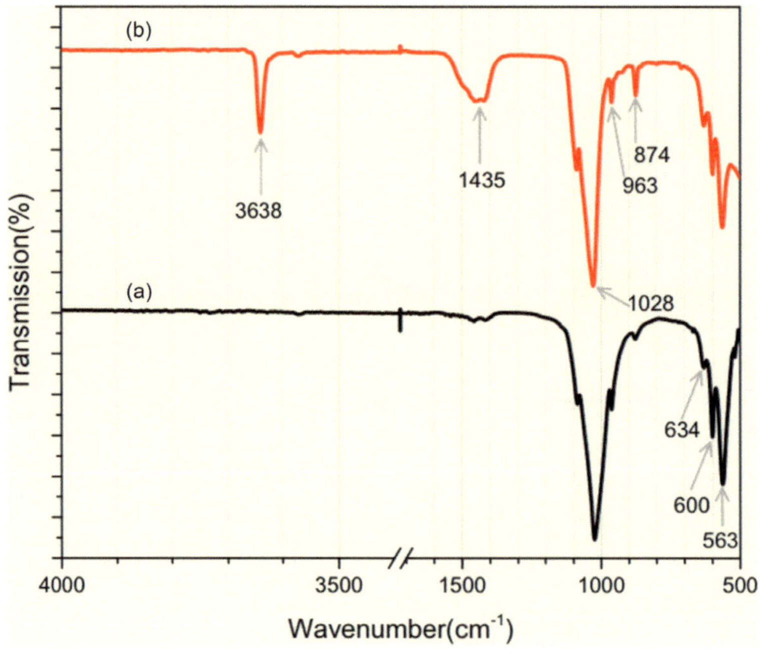

Figure 3.
IR spectra of (a) HAp without heat treatment and (b) HAp with heat treatment at 850°C. The figure is obtained from Asimeng et al.

occur at wavenumbers 1028, 963, 600, and 563 cm^{-1} whereas CO_3^{2-} groups are found at 1435 and 874 cm^{-1}. The HAp is subjected to a temperature of 850°C for 12 h for annealing and normalizing. The heat treatment initiates the substitution of CO_3^{2-} for PO_4^{3-} as indicated in Eq. (4). **Figure 3(b)** shows functional groups of the heat-treated HAp. The CO_3^{2-} groups at 1435 cm^{-1} are now prominent and the OH^- groups, which are absent in HAp without heat treatment, are also intense, which serves as evidence of B-type carbonate HAp.

$$Ca_{10-\frac{x}{2}}(PO_4)_{6-x}(OH)_2 + CO_{3x} \xrightarrow{heattreatment} Ca_{9.5}(PO_4)_5CO_3(OH)_2 \tag{4}$$

5. Discussion

Natural sources for hydroxyapatite synthesis have generated a lot of interest in recent times due to the various advantages it presents over synthetic sources in terms of similarity to the biological apatite (bone and dental). Some of these sources include but are not limited to plants, bovine bone, eggshells, and snail shells. All these biogenic sources have calcium carbonate as a precursor for HAp synthesis. Plant and algae, however, do not have a lot of calcium carbonate as compared to the other sources like bovine, eggshells, and snail shells [19]. The extraction of HAp, therefore, becomes somewhat laborious as there is the need for the addition of more calcium and/or phosphate precursors. This complicated process and the usage of additional calcium or phosphate source increases the cost of production. Clearly, this relegates plant and algae as a great source of HAp for biomedical applications. Biogenic sources such as seashells are rich in $CaCO_3$; however, due to their aquatic nature, they require additional processes/treatment to transform them into a pure phase of HAp [20]. The employment of a combination of extraction methods to achieve the transformation affects the cost of production greatly.

The increasing consumption of snails (Achatina sp.) as a delicacy across all of West Africa has caused a significant increase in snail shell waste production. The recovery of these shells allows for HAp synthesis and reduction in solid wastes. It is recorded in the literature that eggshells and snail shells have a lot of calcium carbonate but the percentage composition in snail shells is more than in eggshells [21]. Snail shells are reported to have about 95–99% calcium carbonate [21]. Bovine bones, comparable to snail shells, present excellent properties to extract HAp but using bovine bones would require a processing technique (hydrothermal process), which is very expensive.

Several extraction methods have been documented for the synthesis of HAp. These fabrication methods include dry methods (solid-state and mechanochemical), wet methods (chemical precipitation, hydrolysis, sol-gel, hydrothermal, emulsion, and sonochemical), and high-temperature processes (combustion and pyrolysis) [22]. It is mostly reported in the literature that wet chemical precipitation tops the chart when it comes to cost-effectiveness considering the materials used and their availability. Also, the use of the wet chemical precipitation method typically results in a low crystalline material compared to a hydrothermally extracted HAp. According to ISO 23317, calcium apatite similar to the bone or enamel apatite should be Ca-deficient and made up of impurities such as CO_3^{2-} and Na^+ and have low crystallinity. It should be noted that for biomedical applications, one desirable property is nano-sized particles. The extraction of nano-sized HAp has advantages in terms of high surface activity and ultrafine structures [23–25], higher bioactivity, and better resorbability than micron-sized particles. With this in mind, the author

Properties	Mammalian (bovine bone, porcine bone, horse bone, camel bone)	Aquatic/marine (fish scales, fish bone)	Other shells (cockle shell, clam, sea shell, eggshell)	Plant/algae	AA shell
Morphology	Irregular, rod-like, flakelike, needle-like, plate-like	Flat-plate, hexagonal, rod-like, irregular, nearly spherical, agglomerate, vary	Spherical, needle-like, rod like, globules, agglomerate polygonal	Flakes, cluster, rectangular, elongate	Needle-like, rod like, spheroids
Particle size	20 nm–500 μm	5 nm–1.0 μm	5 nm–10.4 μm	50–500 nm	12–17 nm
Crystallinity	High (calcination) Low (chemical treatment)	High (calcination) Low (chemical treatment)	High (combination method) Low (chemical treatment)	High (calcination) Low (chemical treatment)	78.2–83.32%
Crystalline Phases	HAp, β-TCP, CaO	HAp, β-TCP, TCP	HAp, calcite, βTCP	HAp þ whitlockite, $CaCO_3$, βTCP, SiO_2	HAp, calcite
References	[26–30]	[31–36]	[37–41]	[42–46]	Asimeng et al.

Table 1.
A summary of the properties of HAp from different biogenic sources.

has successfully extracted HAp from AA shells with particle size in the nanosize range in his previous works. Also, it should be noted that results of an earlier work conducted by Asimeng et al. on the extraction of HAp from the AA shells highlight particle size, lattice parameters, physiochemical properties, and morphological characteristics typical of the human enamel apatite. HAp obtained from the AA shells has further been subjected to a heat treatment to obtain a B-type carbonated HAp and this has significantly improved the physicochemical properties for applications in dentistry and orthopedics. The unit cell parameters of HAp with and without heat treatment are reported by Asimeng et al. The crystallographic information of the B-type carbonated HAp supports the theory that the unit cell a-axis decreases whereas c-axis increases as compared to the HAp without heat treatment.

Table 1 provides a comparative summary of properties of HAp extracted from the different sources and AA shell.

6. Conclusion

This book chapter discussed the synthesis of heat-treated B-type carbonated hydroxyapatite (CHAp) from *Achatina achatina* snail shells and diammonium hydrogen phosphate (DHP) for human calcified tissue replacement and coatings. The synthesis process is in three steps: [1] conversion of the shell crystal structure from aragonite to calcite, [2] precipitation of calcite and DHP to form hydroxyapatite (HAp), and [3] annealing and normalizing the HAp to form B-type CHAp. The synthesis reveals that calcination temperature plays a key role in step [1]. It was noticed that temperatures from 800 to 850°C provided an additional phase (calcium hydroxide) that is required to produce hydroxyl groups for the phosphoric ester formation needed for the HAp synthesis. Also, it is recorded herein that heat treatment facilitated the substitution of CO_3^{2-}.

Acknowledgements

The authors acknowledge Mr. Osman Wahidu and Mr. Richard Asiamah for the support provided during material synthesis.

Author details

Bernard Owusu Asimeng*, David Walter Afeke and Elvis Kwason Tiburu
Department of Biomedical Engineering, University of Ghana, Legon, Ghana

*Address all correspondence to: boasimeng@ug.edu.gh

References

[1] Kannan S, Ventura JM, Ferreira JMF. In situ formation and characterization of flourine-substituted biphasic calcium phosphate ceramics of varied F-HAP/β-TCP ratios. Chemistry of Materials. 2005;**17**(12):3065-3068

[2] Chavan PN, Bahir MM, Mene RU, Mahabole MP, Khairnar RS. Study of nanobiomaterial hydroxyapatite in simulated body fluid: Formation and growth of apatite. Materials Science and Engineering B. 2010;**168**(1):224-230. DOI: 10.1016/j.mseb.2009.11.012

[3] Hui J, Li H, Zheng X, Ma H, Fan D, Liu H, et al. Control synthesis and self-assembly of calcium apatite at low temperatures. Ceramics International [Internet]. 2015;**41**(5):6194-6202. DOI: 10.1016/j.ceramint.2014.12.156

[4] Šimková L, Gorodylova N, Dohnalová Ž, Šulcová P. Influence of precipitation conditions on the synthesis of hydroxyapatite. Ceramics-Silikáty. 2018;**62**(3):253-260

[5] Tayyebi S, Mirjalili F, Samadi H, Nemati A. A review of synthesis and properties of hydroxyapatite / alumina Nano composite powder. Chemistry Journal. 2015;**05**(2):20-28

[6] Yashima M, Yonehara Y, Fujimori H. Experimental visualization of chemical bonding and structural disorder in hydroxyapatite through charge and nuclear-density analysis. Journal of Physical Chemistry C. 2011;**115**(50): 25077-25087

[7] Tank KP, Sharma P, Kanchan DK, Joshi MJ. FTIR, powder XRD, TEM and dielectric studies of pure and zinc doped nano-hydroxyapatite. Crystal Research and Technology. 2011;**46**(12):1309-1316

[8] Dorozhkin SV, Epple M. Biological and medical significance of calcium phosphates. Angewandte Chemie, International Edition. 2002;**41**(12): 3130-3146

[9] Barralet J, Best S, Bonfield W. Carbonate substitution in precipitated hydroxyapatite: An investigation into the effects of reaction temperature and bicarbonate ion concentration. Journal of Biomedical Materials Research. 1998; **41**(1):79-86

[10] Astala R, Stott MJ. First principles investigation of mineral component of bone: CO3 substitutions in hydroxyapatite. Chemistry of Materials. 2005;**17**(16):4125-4133

[11] Landi E, Tampieri A, Mattioli-Belmonte M, Celotti G, Sandri M, Gigante A, et al. Biomimetic Mg- and Mg,CO3-substituted hydroxyapatites: Synthesis characterization and in vitro behaviour. Journal of the European Ceramic Society. 2006;**26**(13): 2593-2601

[12] Ren F, Leng Y. Carbonated apatite, type-a or type-B? Key Engineering Materials. 2012;**493**:293-297

[13] LeGeros RZ. Properties of osteoconductive biomaterials: Calcium phosphates. Clinical Orthopaedics and Related Research. 2002;**395**:81-98

[14] Asimeng BO, Fianko JR, Kaufmann EE, Tiburu EK, Hayford CF, Anani PA, et al. Preparation and characterization of hydroxyapatite from Achatina achatina snail shells: Effect of carbonate substitution and trace elements on defluoridation of water. Journal of Asian Ceramic Societies. 2018;**6**(3):205-212

[15] Madupalli H, Pavan B, Tecklenburg MMJ. Carbonate substitution in the mineral component of bone: Discriminating the structural changes, simultaneously imposed by carbonate in a and B sites of apatite.

Journal of Solid State Chemistry. 2017; **255**:27-35

[16] Zapanta-Legeros R. Effect of carbonate on the lattice parameters of apatite. Nature. 1965;**206**(4982):403-404

[17] Coates J. Interpretation of infrared spectra, a practical approach. Encyclopedia of Analytical Chemistry: Applications, Theory and Instrumentation. 2006

[18] Akram M, Ahmed R, Shakir I, Ibrahim WAW, Hussain R. Extracting hydroxyapatite and its precursors from natural resources. Journal of Materials Science. 2014;**49**(4):1461-1475

[19] Oladele IO, Agbabiaka OG, Olasunkanmi OG, Balogun AO, Popoola MO. Non-synthetic sources for the development of hydroxyapatite. Journal of Applied Biotechnology & Bioengineering. 2018;**5**:92-99

[20] Mohd Pu'ad NAS, Koshy P, Abdullah HZ, Idris MI, Lee TC. Syntheses of hydroxyapatite from natural sources. Heliyon. 2019;**5**(5): e01588

[21] White MM, Chejlava M, Fried B, Sherma J. The concentration of calcium carbonate in shells of freshwater snails. American Malacological Bulletin. 2007; **22**(1):139-142

[22] Zhang X, Vecchio KS. Hydrothermal synthesis of hydroxyapatite rods. Journal of Crystal Growth. 2007;**308**(1): 133-140

[23] Vallet-Regí M, González-Calbet JM. Calcium phosphates as substitution of bone tissues. Progress in Solid State Chemistry. 2004;**32**(1–2):1-31

[24] Cai Y, Liu Y, Yan W, Hu Q, Tao J, Zhang M, et al. Role of hydroxyapatite nanoparticle size in bone cell proliferation. Journal of Materials Chemistry. 2007;**17**(36):3780-3787

[25] Wang J, Burken JG, Zhang XJ. Effect of seeding materials and mixing strength on Struvite precipitation. Water Environment Research. 2006; **78**(2):125-132

[26] Ayatollahi MR, Yahya MY, Asgharzadeh Shirazi H, Hassan SA. Mechanical and tribological properties of hydroxyapatite nanoparticles extracted from natural bovine bone and the bone cement developed by nano-sized bovine hydroxyapatite filler. Ceramics International. 2015;**41**(9): 10818-10827

[27] Ruksudjarit A, Pengpat K, Rujijanagul G, Tunkasiri T. Synthesis and characterization of nanocrystalline hydroxyapatite from natural bovine bone. Current Applied Physics. 2008;**8** (3–4):270-272

[28] Barakat NAM, Khil MS, Omran AM, Sheikh FA, Kim HY. Extraction of pure natural hydroxyapatite from the bovine bones bio waste by three different methods. Journal of Materials Processing Technology. 2009;**209**(7): 3408-3415

[29] Hosseinzadeh E, Davarpanah M, Nemati NH, Tavakoli SA. Fabrication of a hard tissue replacement using natural hydroxyapatite derived from bovine bones by thermal decomposition method. International Journal of Organ Transplantation Medicine. 2014;**5**(1):23

[30] Sun RX, Lv Y, Niu YR, Zhao XH, Cao DS, Tang J, et al. Physicochemical and biological properties of bovine-derived porous hydroxyapatite/collagen composite and its hydroxyapatite powders. Ceramics International [Internet]. 2017;**43**(18):16792-16798. DOI: 10.1016/j.ceramint.2017.09.075

[31] Paul S, Pal A, Choudhury AR, Bodhak S, Balla VK, Sinha A, et al. Effect of trace elements on the sintering effect of fish scale derived hydroxyapatite and its bioactivity.

Ceramics International. 2017;**43**(17): 15678-15684

[32] Pal A, Paul S, Choudhury AR, Balla VK, Das M, Sinha A. Synthesis of hydroxyapatite from lates calcarifer fish bone for biomedical applications. Materials Letters. 2017;**203**:89-92

[33] Sunil BR, Jagannatham M. Producing hydroxyapatite from fish bones by heat treatment. Materials Letters. 2016;**185**:411-414

[34] Pon-On W, Suntornsaratoon P, Charoenphandhu N, Thongbunchoo J, Krishnamra N, Tang IM. Hydroxyapatite from fish scale for potential use as bone scaffold or regenerative material. Materials Science and Engineering: C. 2016;**62**:183-189

[35] Kongsri S, Janpradit K, Buapa K, Techawongstien S, Chanthai S. Nanocrystalline hydroxyapatite from fish scale waste: Preparation, characterization and application for selenium adsorption in aqueous solution. Chemical Engineering Journal. 2013;**215**:522-532

[36] Venkatesan J, Qian ZJ, Ryu B, Thomas NV, Kim SK. A comparative study of thermal calcination and an alkaline hydrolysis method in the isolation of hydroxyapatite from Thunnus obesus bone. Biomedical Materials. 2011;**6**(3):035003

[37] Mustaffa R, Mohd Yusof MR, Abdullah Y. A novelty of synthetic hydroxyapatite from cockle shell and characterization. Advances in Materials Research. 2015;**1087**:429-433

[38] Santhosh S, Balasivanandha PS. Thermal stability of nano hydroxyapatite synthesized from sea shells through wet chemical synthesis. Materials Letters. 2013;**19**:121-124

[39] Mohamad Razali NAI, Pramanik S, Abu Osman NA, Radzi Z, Pingguan-Murphy B. Conversion of calcite from cockle shells to bioactive nanorod hydroxyapatite for biomedical applications. Journal of Ceramic Processing Research. 2016;**17**:699-706

[40] Pal A, Maity S, Chabri S, Bera S, Chowdhury AR, Das M, et al. Mechanochemical synthesis of nanocrystalline hydroxyapatite from Mercenaria clam shells and phosphoric acid. Biomedical Physics & Engineering Express. 2017;**3**(1):015010

[41] Goloshchapov DL, Kashkarov VM, Rumyantseva NA, Seredin PV, Lenshin AS, Agapov BL, et al. Synthesis of nanocrystalline hydroxyapatite by precipitation using hen's eggshell. Ceramics International. 2013;**39**(4): 4539-4549

[42] Govindaraj D, Rajan M. Synthesis and spectral characterization of novel nano-hydroxyapatite from Moringaoleifera leaves. Materials Today: Proceedings. 2016;**3**(6):2394-2398

[43] Tampieri A, Sprio S, Ruffini A, Celotti G, Lesci IG, Roveri N. From wood to bone: Multi-step process to convert wood hierarchical structures into biomimetic hydroxyapatite scaffolds for bone tissue engineering. Journal of Materials Chemistry. 2009; **12**(28):4973-4980

[44] Monballiu A, Desmidt E, Ghyselbrecht K, Meesschaert B. Phosphate recovery as hydroxyapatite from nitrified UASB effluent at neutral pH in a CSTR. Journal of Environmental Chemical Engineering. 2018;**6**(4): 4413-4422

[45] Teymouri A, Stuart BJ, Kumar S. Hydroxyapatite and dittmarite precipitation from algae hydrolysate. Algal Research. 2018;**29**:202-211

[46] Tsuru K, Ruslin, Maruta M, Matsuya S, Ishikawa K. Effects of the method of apatite seed crystals addition on setting reaction of α-tricalcium phosphate based apatite cement. Journal of Materials Science. Materials in Medicine. 2015;**26**(10):244

Chapter 7

Innovative Hybrid Materials with Improved Tensile Strength Obtained by 3D Printing

Roxana Mioara Piticescu, Laura Madalina Cursaru, Gabriela Negroiu, Cristina Florentina Ciobota, Ciprian Neagoe and Daniel Safranchik

Abstract

Barium titanate (BT) and barium strontium titanate (BST) are one of the most studied ferroelectric materials with excellent piezoelectric properties, which can be used to stimulate bone formation by applying an electrical field. It is known that this ceramic is biocompatible and can be used for medical applications. New hybrid materials based on BT and collagen and BST and collagen, with potential applications in bone reconstruction, are presented, emphasizing the potential of fabricating 3D structures by integrating hydrothermal synthesis with additive manufacturing. Designing such structures may take advantage of rheological characterization at single-molecule level for some elastic biopolymers like titin and collagen and their molecular dissection into structural motifs that independently contribute to the protein viscoelasticity. Atomic force spectroscopy measurements on synthetic polypeptides showed that a polypeptide chain containing Ig domain modules is protected against rupture at high stretch by Ig domain unfolding, an important mechanism for stress relaxation in titin molecules. This property may be exploited to enhance the tensile strength of a 3D structure by adding specific synthetic polypeptides to the composition of the printing paste.

Keywords: barium titanate, barium strontium titanate, 3D printing, titin, Ig domain, fracture mechanics

1. Introduction

Bone defects occur due to malformations, traumatic lesions, and tumor resections. Biomaterials for bone defect reconstruction consist of osteosynthetic materials that are placed in the cavity left behind by osteotomies or traumatic lesions. Other applications refer to dental implants with functional or aesthetic role in the facial region. The results of bone reconstruction are dependent on the surgical skills, the quality of the adjacent tissue, the size and location of the bone defect, as well as the method of repairing the bone defect. Current methods of reconstruction include simple or vascularized bone grafts, the use of biomaterials, and, more recently, the use of growth factors to induce osteoinduction [1].

The use of autologous bone for orthopedic reconstruction may be restricted due to the limited amount of donor bone from the sampling areas. It is possible that the bone tissue taken may require reshaping into custom shapes, which may complicate the surgical operation. Also, complications in the case of simple bone grafts include graft resorption and increased mortality associated with the sampling area [1].

The benefits of alloplastic materials have been reported in the literature, being used as such or in combination with bone transplants or osteoinductive cytokines. The procedure can be used not only to replace the missing bone but also to stimulate osteoinduction, acting as a scaffold material for bone regeneration. The implanted materials should be biocompatible, without any side effects or toxicity. However, over time complications and toxicities of implanted biomaterials used in orthopedic surgery have been reported, often leading to inflammation associated with leukocytosis and fibrosis.

For osteosynthesis, titanium alloy prostheses offer major advantages in terms of biocompatibility, stability, and individual implant placement. Removal of asymptomatic prostheses and screws after fracture healing is still controversial due to the fact that the removal procedure could damage the bone [1].

The large variety of biomaterials for bone defect reconstruction makes it difficult to choose the right material for surgical areas and specific applications. An optimal biomaterial meets all the requirements: biocompatibility, stability, intraoperative matching, product safety, and low costs; in reality, the perfect material has not yet been found. The development of future materials aims to improve the physical and biological properties, especially regarding surface interactions [1].

While the popularity of hydroxyapatite-based ceramic materials as filler for critical bone defects is known in the community of specialists in bioengineering, materials science, and orthopedic and dental surgery, only a few studies address piezoelectric materials for bone regeneration, such as barium titanate (BT) [$BaTiO_3$] and barium strontium titanate (BST) [$Ba_{0.7}Sr_{0.3}TiO_3$]. The potential effect of this class of materials in bone tissue engineering is due to its dielectric properties, low dielectric loss, and polarization. Sr^{2+} ion can increase a dielectric constant, and it is a trace element in the human body that plays a dual role in bone formation and regeneration [2].

On the other hand, barium titanate-based ceramic with perovskite structure has been widely used as a ferroelectric material for its attractive properties, such as high piezoelectric coefficient (d_{33} = 191 pC/N) as well as excellent biocompatibility and bone regeneration capacity in the complex physiological environment, and is further considered as an intelligent material for tissue reconstruction [2–4].

Since 1954, it has been reported that natural bone is a piezoelectric material [5–12]. In 1957, Fukada et al. [8] observed that the stress-induced piezoelectric effect in bone was due to the slipping of collagen fibers past one another. The bone tissue exhibited a very low piezoelectric coefficient of 0.7 pC/N [13] and was demonstrated to be biologically active and would respond to micromechanical stress such as the movement of the body itself, leading to the generation of an electrical dipole [14, 15]. Piezoelectric materials can provide the electrical stimulation characteristic for natural bone environment as it has been asserted that bone growth and repair are promoted by the electrical signals produced when the bone is mechanically stressed [16]. Due to their parallel features with the real bone, piezoelectric materials for bone tissue reconstruction may become the next generation of bone grafts [17]. Piezoelectric property of barium titanate could be used as a charge supply to stimulate the bone implant healing process. So far, all the piezoelectric ceramics used in vivo and vitro were in the dense bulk form [18]. However, owing to the interconnected pores to provide a favorable environment for bone ingrowth and osseointegration [19], a functional bone implant should be porous [15], to create strong bonds with the host natural tissue by allowing cellular penetration and encouraging new cells for tissue regeneration.

One of the best ways to achieve this goal is to use an osteoconductive and porous structure to act as a three-dimensional (3D) porous scaffold [2]. Ideally, osseointegration of the grafted material would be accomplished on a long timescale by the progressive action of osteoclasts, osteoblasts, and osteocytes which remove the graft material and deposit new bone in place [20]. Having a structure that resembles the natural design and composition may not always respond to functional requirements of a medical application. Bioresorbable scaffolds to replace bone defects must have a high porosity—a pore size of 50–800 μm—to allow the infiltration of cells and nutrients into the implant [21]; the porosity of the material should accommodate new osteon growth, requiring 200 μm pore size, to allow growth of new capillaries, optimal for 50 μm pore size, whereas interconnected micropores lower than 10 μm improve the metabolic environment and fluid circulation through capillarity [22]. The apparent conflicting requirements are met with a 3D design that does not correspond to the natural structure of the bone. Furthermore, improving the osmotic or mechanical properties of the synthetic bone graft material by adding components that are not present in the natural bone may address the needs of some common bone diseases like osteoporosis [23], where graft resorption and replacement by native bone tissue may not be the best option.

In recent years, the development of 3D printing techniques for the manufacture of ceramic-based scaffold materials has shown promising outcomes [1, 2].

Bioprinting technologies have grown rapidly in the last decade, being also known as "additive manufacturing" or "extrusion bioprinting." Bioprinting can be defined as a spatial method of stratified deposition of a biological material (or support for biological material), based on a computerized, layer-by-layer model, using a CAD-CAM system.

The structure of the computerized model can be modified and rearranged with the passage of each layer, so as to obtain a complex final model that mimics the tissue structure. The versatility of the technology allows the adoption of an unlimited number of material combinations for extrusion, thus ensuring the possibility of developing unique three-dimensional models, adapted from case to case. Extrusion bioprinting technology is a combination of an automated robotic system, controlled by software and an extrusion distribution system of the material in the custom 3D structure. This process ensures speed but also structural integrity due to the computerized continuous deposition system. 3D models can be obtained, generated, imported, and exported from any CAD system, including data obtained from medical imaging systems such as computer tomography (CT) and/or nuclear magnetic resonance (NMR). The material deposition system can be operated by means of a screw mechanism and stepper motor, pneumatically, by piston-compressed air mechanism, or by solenoid-electromagnetic system. Deposition systems by screw mechanism are more precise, can be better controlled, and also provide controlled deposition in the case of very viscous substances. These deposition systems can be assembled on a 3D bioprinting machine so that they work in synergy, especially if two different materials are deposited. Unlike other additive manufacturing processes, extrusion bioprinting does not require large amounts of energy and is an environmentally friendly method. In addition it has a high standardization capacity and does not require special auxiliary installations. A characteristic is that it can produce, under specific conditions, materials with a porous structure and shape similar to the anatomical one, likely to attain biocompatibility status.

The 3D printing technique allows the manufacturing of scaffold-type materials with complex internal structures and high resolution, designed according to the specific needs of each patient. The technology of extruding materials in the form of pastes, which are passed through a nozzle or hole to obtain fibers arranged as three-dimensional structures of different shapes, is suitable for the manufacture of hard tissue scaffolds in bone tissue engineering.

Scaffolds are of utmost importance in tissue engineering because they provide the necessary support for cell proliferation and differentiation. Also, the scaffold's architecture defines the final form of the new organ. Biocompatibility of scaffolds made by 3D printing, as well as different aspects of their interaction with cells, has been explored in numerous studies by in vitro and in vivo tests [21].

The extrusion-based additive manufacturing techniques are favorable for printing scaffold structures due to the ability to process a wide range of biomaterials with controlled porosity and to generate interconnected pores, which represent essential requirements for cell growth [22]. The topography of the surface of the biomaterial as well as its architecture on the micro- and nanoscale plays an important role in bone tissue engineering. Cao et al. have shown increased tissue regeneration and decreased inflammatory reactions in the case of aligned fiber scaffolds, compared to scaffolds whose fibers were randomly arranged [24].

Regarding 3D printing of barium titanate (BT) ceramics for medical applications, Schult et al. [25], have shown that BT powder can serve as a material for bone reconstruction, obtained by 3D printing cylindrical parts with 11.7 mm in diameter and 3.51 mm high, out of the three BT-based mixtures. The first mixture, M1, consisted of untreated BT powder, a stable polymer, and a flow additive—AEROSIL R8200. The second mixture, M2, has the same composition as the first, but BT was previously subjected to a heat treatment of calcination, using for this a fraction of the sieved powder of 60–80 μm and a flow additive. The third mixture, M3, also contains calcined BT, but in this case the fractions <125 μm and 125–250 μm were used in a ratio of 1:2, without adding flow additives, because the powder has good fluidity. To bond the material, a soluble polymer granulate with a mean grain size of 50 μm was used in all three mixtures. Solupor-Binder (Voxeljet AG, Germany) is used as a binder fluid. The binder partially dissolves the polymer granulate so that the ceramic particles glue together. The porosity was visible in all samples, being beneficial for cell growth. After sintering, the largest contraction was observed in the case of the M1 sample, of 75.53%, but the other two also recorded relatively high contractions, M2 of 40.55% and M3 of 29.51%. The results reported in their study confirm that porous barium titanate ceramics can be used as a 3D structure for bone tissue engineering and bone formation can be promoted by electrical stimulation [25].

In other study, a binder jetting additive manufacturing technology was used to fabricate robust geometric barium titanate specimens of $12 \times 12 \times 3$ mm^3 by using commercial BT powder [26]. The results presented in their work have shown that 3D printing allows the manufacture of custom, conformal, geometrically complex piezoelectric devices for next-generation industries such as biomedical ones. One example includes the possibility of an energy-harvesting active biomedical implant, the shape of which could be customized for patient-specific geometry corresponding to anatomical features and use (e.g., a bone implant that will eliminate the need for battery replacement and resulting follow-on surgeries).

2. Design of multilayered ceramic materials

Fractures occur in ceramics as a result of crack propagation. The science of design against fractures is based on the pioneering work of A.A. Griffith (1893– 1963) who proposed an energy balance approach to predict fracture strengths in materials [27]. Thus, crack growth is associated with the release of strain energy and absorption of energy to create the two flanking surfaces. In a succinct manner, we may calculate the stress level σ_f when crack propagation occurs using the Griffith equation:

$$\sigma_f = \sqrt{\frac{2E\gamma}{\pi a}}, \tag{1}$$

where E is the Young modulus, γ is the surface energy, and a is the size of the crack or defect. This describes well very brittle materials, which do not exhibit plasticity domains before fracture. A more general description was developed based on the original Griffith equation by Irwin [28] and Orowan [29] as follows:

$$\sigma_f = \sqrt{\frac{E\varsigma_c}{\pi a}}, \tag{2}$$

where critical strain release rate parameter, ς_c, was introduced to consider the energy dissipation into material due to a ductile behavior of the material. A more detailed description of the problem is provided by Roylance [30].

The design of fracture-resistant materials by combining viscoelastic polymers with ceramic materials would be either as composites (separate components) or in the form of mixtures. A composite beam made of multiple layers of ceramics interrupted by polymer layers would be protected against catastrophic crack propagation across layers. Based on the Griffith energy balance approach, it is possible to find out the ceramic layer thickness that would maximize fracture resistance. Griffith equation was historically used to describe fracture resistance dependency on grain size (d_{grain}) in carbon steel and thus explain some catastrophic failures of low-grade steels at temperature transitions. At plastic to brittle transition of the material, the crack was considered to propagate along the whole grain and dissipate at grain boundaries. Replacing $a = d_{grain}$ in Eq. (2), it results:

$$\sigma_f = \text{v}\sqrt{\frac{E\varsigma_c}{\pi\, d_{grain}}}, \tag{3}$$

Analogously, for a multilayered ceramic material (**Figure 1**) shaped as a beam with equally thick longitudinal layers, we plot fracture stress against layer thickness, considering the most unfavorable situation when the crack expands immediately across the whole layer. The relative units refer to maximal fracture stress and beam thickness for normalization. From the fracture stress curve, it results, at a first view, that very thin layers would provide the beam with maximal protection against fractures. Another criterion for optimization is provided by efficiency reasoning.

Subjected to tensile stress, the beam would distribute the load on individual layers according to their thickness. A maximal fracture-proof design of a multilayered beam would consider that even a single layer would be able to support the whole beam load, meaning that the tension applied on the layer is lower than the beam fracture tension. Intuitively, a beam consisting of two layers is a minimal backup mechanism, whereas more layers may look excessive for most applications. In the graph in **Figure 1**, the intersection between the two curves occurs for a number of 10 layers. In other words, for a beam designed to resist fracture, more than 10 layers would not provide reliance on single layer last standing (the initial premise), whereas less than this number lowers the fracture-safe tension limit. Therefore 10 longitudinal ceramic layers, uncoupled for fracture propagation, may already provide the safest design for tensile load fractures in a beam. The underlying supposition is that the ultimate tensile strength has the same order of magnitude as the fracture strength. Transversal loads on the beam would require a change in the design of the multilayered beam; still the reasoning example for longitudinal loads demonstrates how to look for the optimal grain size in order to

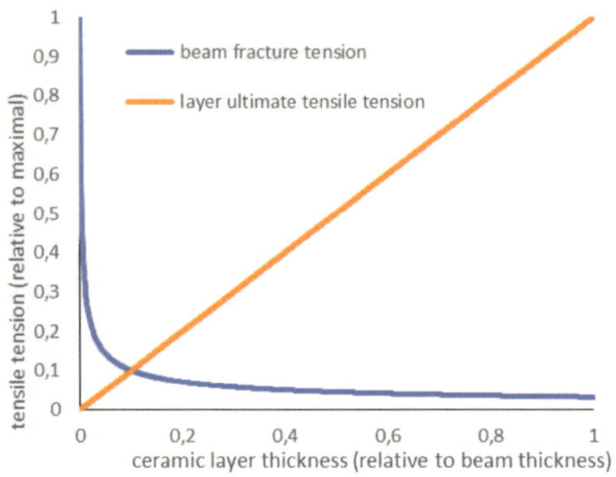

Figure 1.
A proposed criterion for fracture-proof layer thickness in layered beams made of brittle ceramics exposed to longitudinal stretch. Intersection between curves describing ultimate tensile tension of a layer (orange), and beam fracture tension (blue) provides a point of optimal layer thickness to stand alone against the whole beam stretch load.

build fracture-resistant polymer-reinforced ceramic materials. Thus, decreasing the grain size to nanometer level does not bring additional fracture resistance to millimeter-thick ceramic objects. The 3D printed material in **Figure 5** is made of ceramic-collagen filaments ~0.6 mm thick oriented in two perpendicular directions and connected in the nodes. The filaments are made of globular grains 2–10 μm in diameter. This structure actually relies on the binder to hold the grains together. The space between grains is large enough to accommodate biopolymer filaments as binder; one way to produce such filaments in place is to populate the spongy structure with fibroblasts and grow them in culture, as we show here. Then a weak link will reside inside ceramic-polymer hybrid grains.

3. Ceramic-polymer hybrid materials

Adding a polymer to a ceramic material in 3D printing is in the first place a mean to modulate the viscosity of the printing paste and support complex 3D structures while they are raised by adding material. Keeping the polymer in place or removing it by post-processing of the printed object depends on the contribution of the polymer to the mechanical properties of the printed object. The brittleness of glasses and ceramic materials is usually addressed by reinforcing the brittle material with elastic fibers, either as composite or as mixture. In mixtures, nanoscale contact between ceramic materials and polymers intimately modulates the elasticity of the resulting material. Aragonite and hydroxyapatite have a very high elastic modulus, around 100 GPa, and a fracture toughness of ~1 $MPa/m^{1/2}$. With those values, based on some common assumptions, Chen et al. estimated [31] that the brittleness domain of the material is in the nanometer range. Biological structures based on aragonite (nacre) or hydroxyapatite (like bones) rely on elastic biopolymers as binders to increase their fracture resistance by dissipating the stress energy. Irwin and Orowan approach on fracture propagation assumes that stress energy is dissipated around fracture tip by plastic deformations, in which a purely entropic polymer does not accomplish. A mechanism for plastic deformations in nacre resides in micrometer-sized parallel platelets that are able to slide on each other. In this case, the binder breaks and forms attachments to the aragonite platelets while the stress is dissipated. This occurs at a micrometer range. On a nanometer scale, viscoelasticity inside the binding biopolymer may provide another mechanism for stress relaxation.

The idea of mixing collagen and ceramic powder in a paste for printing bone grafts or other bone-like structures for medical applications is based on similarity with the natural bone. Ideally, osseointegration of the grafted material would be accomplished on a long timescale by the progressive action of osteoclasts and osteoblasts which remove the graft material and deposit new bone in place. Having a structure that resembles the natural design may not always respond to functional requirements of a medical application. For example, the porosity of the material should accommodate new osteon growth, requiring 200 μm pore size, to allow growth of new capillaries, optimal for 50 μm pore size, whereas interconnected micropores lower than 10 μm improve the metabolic environment and fluid circulation through capillarity [32]. In a mixture, the viscoelastic polymer should significantly add toughness to effectively dissipate strain energy from initiating cracks in ceramics. A relevant group of biological polymers are the proteins involved in the elasticity of animal tissues. An impressive coordinated effort was made to understand the contribution of the giant protein titin to the elasticity of the striated muscle, detailed on structural, mechanical, and enzymatic description of the functional segments in titin molecules. A comprehensive review on the subject is provided by Prof. Wolfgang A. Linke [33].

The Ig domains in titin were described for their viscoelastic role, protecting titin from breaking under excessive stretch. In 1996, Improta, Politou, and Pastore determined the structure of I27 titin Ig domain by nuclear magnetic resonance (NMR) techniques [34]. The I27 titin Ig domain structure consists in two β sheets packing against each other, each β sheet containing four β strands. Stretch-induced unfolding of the Ig structure provides significant additional extension to the titin molecule, as demonstrated by Linke and Fernandez laboratories [35, 36]. Atomic force microscopy of single molecules was used to investigate synthetic polypeptides based on repetitive Ig domain gene constructs.

In **Figure 2** we replotted from literature some AFM force spectroscopy measurements on collagen I molecules [37], a synthetic polypeptide fragment made of 8 repetitive I27 titin Ig domains [38] and a synthetic protein made of repetitive modules found in dragline spider silk protein (16 SPI and 4 SPII modules) [39]. Extension of collagen molecule in the nanometer range generates almost no force, starting to rise at 300 nm extension. Instead, a single I27 module already provides

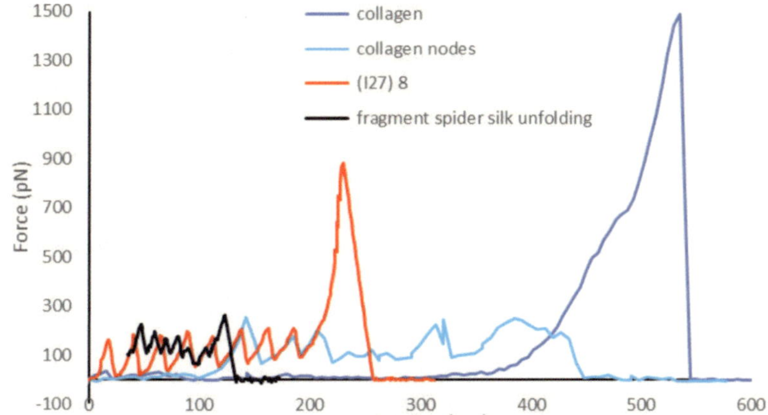

Figure 2.
Comparison of force extension AFM measurements in collagen I single molecules (blue), collagen I interconnected molecules (light blue), a synthetic polypeptide made of 8 repeats of I27 titin Ig module (red) and a synthetic protein fragment made of repetitive modules from dragline spider silk protein (black). Replotted and adapted from Linke et al. for (I27)8 [38], Bozec and Horton [37] for collagen I, and Oroudjev et al. [39] for modular recombinant protein from spider silk.

maximal tension of folded state with 28.1 nm stretch and then unfolds and releases a strain (red line). Unfolding and full extension of all 8 I27 repeats in the polypeptide occurs at ~230 nm stretch, raising the force to 882 pN, which is 59% of the maximal single molecule collagen force. Stretching multiple collagen molecules, as they are connected by nodes in a net, also fails to deliver significant force at nanometer range extensions (light blue line). For comparison, a synthetic recombinant modular fragment from dragline spider silk protein is shown to unfold its modules with a repetitive pattern of 14 nm (black line), releasing lower levels of tension than Ig domain unfolding or collagen I molecule node detachment.

Addition of long-range acting binders (developing significant force only at high extensions) versus short-range acting binders in the composition of hybrid polymer-ceramic material is not an obvious decision. Increasing collagen I molecule concentration would raise the number of cross-links between molecules, thus enabling significant force development at lower extensions (as shown in **Figure 2**, light blue line). Ultimately, as concentration is increased, collagen I molecules will assemble in fibrils with high strength and low extensibility ropelike structures, 260–410 nm wide [40]. This will increase the interspacing between mineral grains or tiles to sizes often found in the natural reign of such materials [41]. Mechanical measurements (indentation technique) on collagen fibrils (50–200 nm in diameter) dissected from rat tail showed a Young elastic modulus in the range from 5 GPa to 11.5 GPa (in air, at room temperature) [42], a value at most 1/10 of hydroxyapatite modulus. The concept is that collagen fibers contribute less to the elastic stiffness of the bone and more to its capacity to absorb deformation energy before it fails, that is, toughness [41]. As part of the energy dissipation of the deformative load, the bone structure suffers plastic deformations at the microstructural level, and, in living organisms, it is repaired and even remodeled to withstand the new actual load configuration. If we consider that natural structures evolved to optimize functionality, then it is important to understand that optimization also means maximal toughness or the solution had to deal with limitations and constrains of the cellular machineries that build bone-like biopolymer-mineral structures.

4. 3D printing of ceramic-polymer hybrid materials

Patient-specific design of orthopedic prosthetic devices may improve the durability and the performance of the device by adequate distribution of loads and by using wear-resistant materials on highly solicited spots. An example is hip arthroplasty where bearings may be adequately designed and fabricated to minimize surface friction between elements [43]. With the use of numerical models, the shape and mechanical properties of the prosthesis could be optimized according to patient characteristics like height, weight, gender, and age. Then, the prosthesis has to be engineered for a suitable mounting procedure during the orthopedic intervention and manufactured according to specifications. Some design features like 3D shape may be attained with standard manufacturing techniques, and other features, particularly those involving material microstructure, are possible only by advanced manufacturing. 3D printing combines the advantage of using directly the results of numerical modeling to create the prosthetic device—eliminating some intermediate steps, with the micrometer precision and versatility of the printing mechanism and allowing for microstructuring and the use of various materials for the same piece.

An example of ceramic-polymer hybrid material fabricated by 3D printing method is presented. *For the first time*, 3D hybrid organic-inorganic materials based on barium titanate and collagen (BTC) and barium strontium titanate and collagen (BST-C), with potential applications as filler in bone tissue engineering, have been

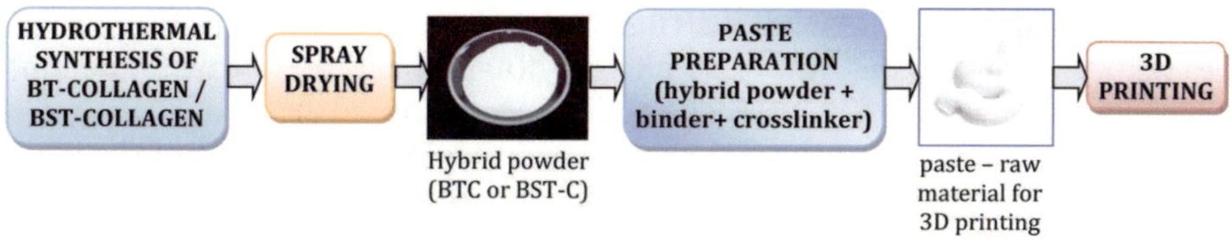

Figure 3.
Technological flow for the fabrication of 3D structures.

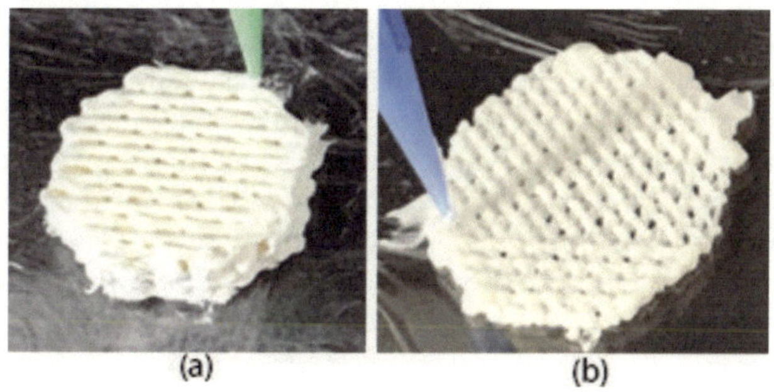

Figure 4.
3D printed scaffolds using two types of nozzles: (a) Ø 0.8 mm (BST-C structure) and (b) Ø 0.4 mm (BTC structure).

developed by extrusion-based 3D printing method, as presented below. Thus, hybrid nanostructured powders (BTC and BST-C) were obtained by the hydrothermal process at high pressure, starting from $Ba(OH)_2*8H_2O$ powder, aqueous solution of TiO_2Cl_2, and collagen powder as BTC precursors and $Ba(OH)_2*8H_2O$ powder, aqueous solution of $Sr(NO_3)_2$, aqueous solution of TiO_2Cl_2, and collagen powder as BST-C precursors. After the solution pH was adjusted at pH > 10, and the hybrid suspension thus prepared was transferred to the Berghof autoclave (Germany) and subjected to hydrothermal synthesis at T < 100°C and p = 40 bar for 2 h. Afterwards, the hybrid nanostructured powders were filtered and washed with distilled water until neutral pH was reached and further spray-dried using a LabPLANT SD-06 spray dryer (UK).

Powders resulted after hydrothermal synthesis were mechanically mixed with a water-soluble polymer binder (Mowiflex, Kuraray Poval) 20% solution and a cross-linking agent (Baymedix® FD103, Covestro), obtaining a viscous paste which is further used as a feedstock in the 3D printing process using 3D BioScaffolder system (SYS-ENG, Germany) equipped with BioScaffolder software (SW) 3.0. The technological flow is briefly depicted in **Figure 3** (synthesis of hybrid powders, preparation of paste, and 3D printing of hybrid structures).

Some examples of 3D hybrid structures obtained with different nozzles and rotation angles between 2 successive layers (90° and 45°, respectively) are given in **Figure 4**.

5. Manufacture of 3D structures based on barium titanate and collagen and barium strontium titanate and collagen by 3D printing method

3D printing is a highly versatile technique to fabricate complex structures with high precision and nanometer resolution. The principle of this technique is based on the extrusion of continuous filaments (inks) in a layer-by-layer sequence using computer-aided design (CAD) tools. This method is capable of fabricating structures with feature sizes on the microscale (0.1–100 μm) and mesoscale (>100 μm), depending on the nozzle diameter. The ability to fabricate a variety of structures requires a good control over the formulation and rheological behavior of the inks and the printing parameters (velocity printing, pressure extrusion). The fundamental advantage for any lattice structure are that it is self-supporting (to bear on itself) without the need for inside supports. Another key aspect for the use of porous structures is pore interconnectivity. Porosity is defined as the total percentage of bare spaces in a solid and is a morphological property independent of the material.

The 3D structures were obtained as described above, using the 3D printing technique and BioScaffolder (SYS-ENG, Germany) device, connected via a USB port to a computer on which the BioScaffolder SW 3.0 software is installed. This software allows the configuration of the 3D object to be created in this program or imported from a CAD-CAM program, as well as the setting of the printing process parameters for the 3D object (scaffold), made by depositing several layers of extruded fibers. The shape of 3D structure can be also set using BioScaffolder software. Thus, cubic, octagonal, and cylindric shapes can be obtained.

6. Morpho-structural characterization of 3D structures

BTC and BST-C structures fabricated as described above have been characterized using different techniques: scanning electron microscopy coupled with energy dispersive X-ray analysis (SEM/EDX), X-ray diffraction (XRD), and optical profilometry.

SEM/EDX analysis was performed using a FEI E-SEM Quanta 200 microscope equipped with EDX. XRD analysis was performed using a Rigaku MiniFlex 2 diffractometer. Optical profilometry measurements were performed using Veeco WYKO NT1100.

6.1 SEM/EDX characterization

SEM images of two representative samples (BTCM-1 and BST-C1) are depicted in **Figures 5** and **6**.

Figure 5b shows a typical image of a 3D structure with fibers having thickness of 512–587 μm, while the distance between them varies between 762 and 1093 μm. **Figure 5a** clearly shows how the fibers are arranged in multiple layers in the 3D structure. The round-shaped particles of barium titanate-based nanopowders can be observed in **Figure 7c**, as a result of $BaTiO_3$ spray-drying.

In the case of BST-C1 sample, the porosity of the structure can be observed in **Figure 6a** (cross section). The fiber thickness varies between 860 and 1064 μm,

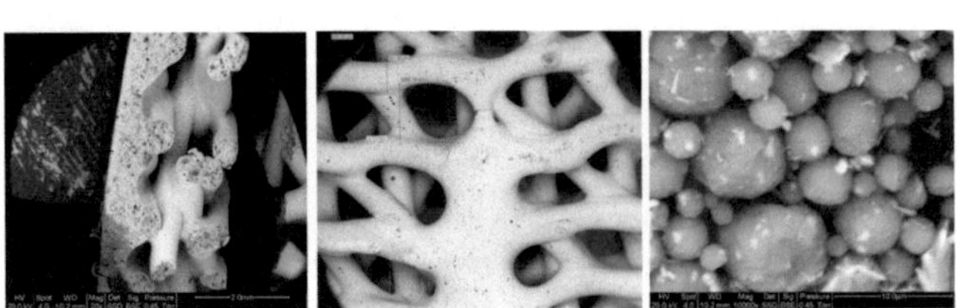

Figure 5.
SEM images of BTCM sample: (a) cross section of 3D sample; (b) front image at 20×; (c) front image at a higher magnification—10,000×.

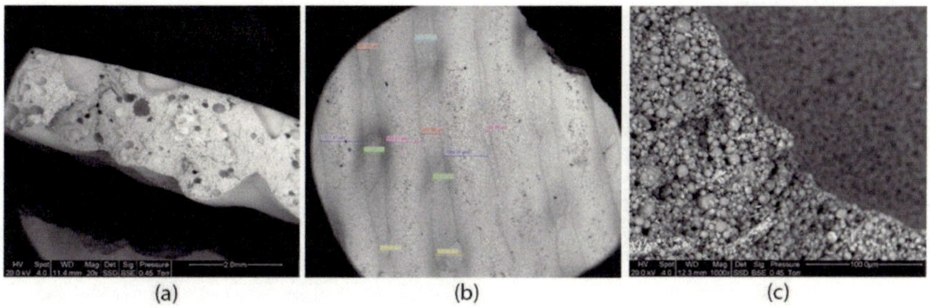

Figure 6.
SEM images of BST-C1 sample: (a) cross section of 3D sample; (b) front image at 33×; (c) front image at a higher magnification—1000×

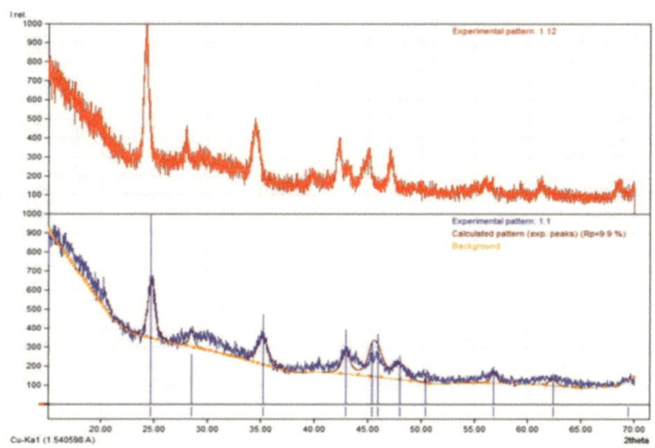

Figure 7.
XRD spectra of BTCM-1.12 sample (in red) and BST-C1.1 sample (in blue).

Sample	C	O	Ti	Ba	Sr	Total
BTCM-1	9.04	29.59	25.37	36.01	—	100.00
BST-C1	14.22	26.50	10.78	8.42	40.09	100.00

Table 1.
Semiquantitative analysis of two representative 3D structures (BTCM and BST-C).

while the distance between them is about 105–543 μm (**Figure 6b**). Similar with BTCM-1 sample, spherical particles of $Ba_xSr_{1-x}TiO_3$ nanopowders are observed in **Figure 6c**. EDX analysis is presented in **Table 1**.

6.2 XRD characterization

XRD spectra of two representative samples (BTCM-1 and BST-C1) are presented in **Figure 7**. From **Figure 7**, it can be seen that the main characteristic peak of $BaTiO_3$ in sample BTCM-1 corresponds to $2\theta = 39.71$ and interplanar distance $d = 2.268$. The crystallite size related to this peak is 14.1 nm, and it was calculated using Scherrer equation. In the case of BST-C1 sample, the main characteristic peak appears at $2\theta = 35.18$ and interplanar distance $d = 2.549$. The crystallite size calculated for this peak using Scherrer equation is 8.9 nm. As it can be seen on the diffraction spectra, non-doped barium titanate (BTCM-1) and Sr-doped barium titanate (BST-C1) powders are slightly shifted. Peak locations are not exactly

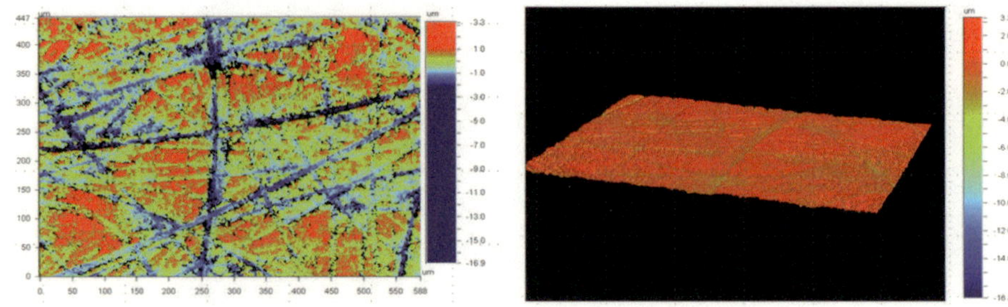

Figure 8.
Surface roughness of BTCM-1.5 sample.

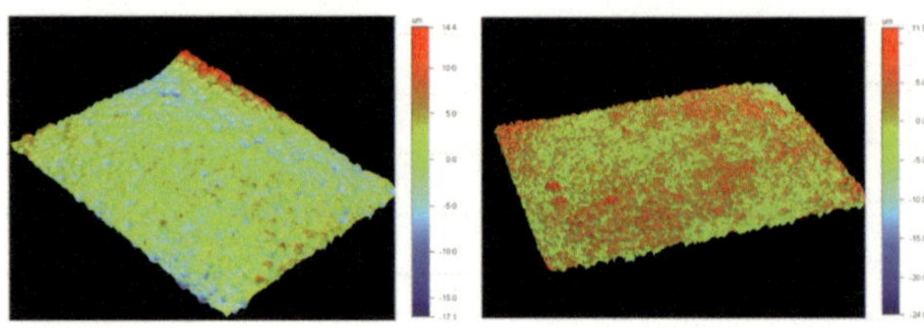

Figure 9.
Surface roughness of BST-C1.3 sample.

suitable to PDF cards of $BaTiO_3$ and $Ba_xSr_{1-x}TiO_3$, which might be explained by the presence of binder and collagen in the powder compositions.

6.3 Optical profilometry

Surface roughness of two representative samples (BTCM-1.5 and BST-C1.3) is depicted in **Figures 8** and **9**. The mean surface roughness Ra (the average roughness of the surface) of BTCM-1.5 is about 600 nm.

The mean surface roughness Ra (the average roughness of the surface) of BST-C1.3 is about 2.29 μm.

7. The stability and biocompatibility of BTCM 3D printed materials for in vitro tests

The BTCM materials were sterilized by immersion for 4 h in an 8 ml sterile phosphate buffer containing 1% penicillin/streptomycin and 0.25 mg/ml amphotericin B (Fungizone) and then washed three times with an 8 ml of sterile phosphate buffer to remove the excess of Fungizone and penicillin/streptomycin. After 4 h of sterilization, the BTCM material retains its structure almost intact and can be handled with care in the next steps. The residues released from BTCM materials at the end of the sterilization period were undetectable visually and demonstrated the biomaterial stability in phosphate buffer. After sterilization the materials to be analyzed were moved into an 8 ml completely sterile DMEM culture medium and kept for 24 h in the incubator at 37°C. This step intended to analyze the impact of the soluble compounds released by the materials, if any, in the cell culture medium on cell morphology and adhesion. The DMEM medium resulted from the 24 h of incubation with BTCM materials was further used for culturing 1070Sk CCD fibroblasts and SKMel23 metastatic melanoma cells. The CCD fibroblasts (passage 23) and SKMel23 melanoma cells (passage 3) were seeded in a cell culture six-well plate at a density of 2×10^4 cells/well, cultured in DMEM medium (control) or DMEM medium resulted from incubation with BTCM materials, for 24 h, and analyzed in bright-field microscopy. The fibroblasts grown in the DMEM medium exposed to the BTCM material were completely adhered to the substrate and had a morphology similar to the controls (**Figure 10**). In the case of SkMel23 cells grown in DMEM exposed to BTCM material, the cells also well adhered to the substrate. However, their morphology was slightly different compared to the control cells (**Figure 11**). Next we investigated whether SkMel23 cells were able to adhere to the BTCM material itself. For this purpose, a suspension

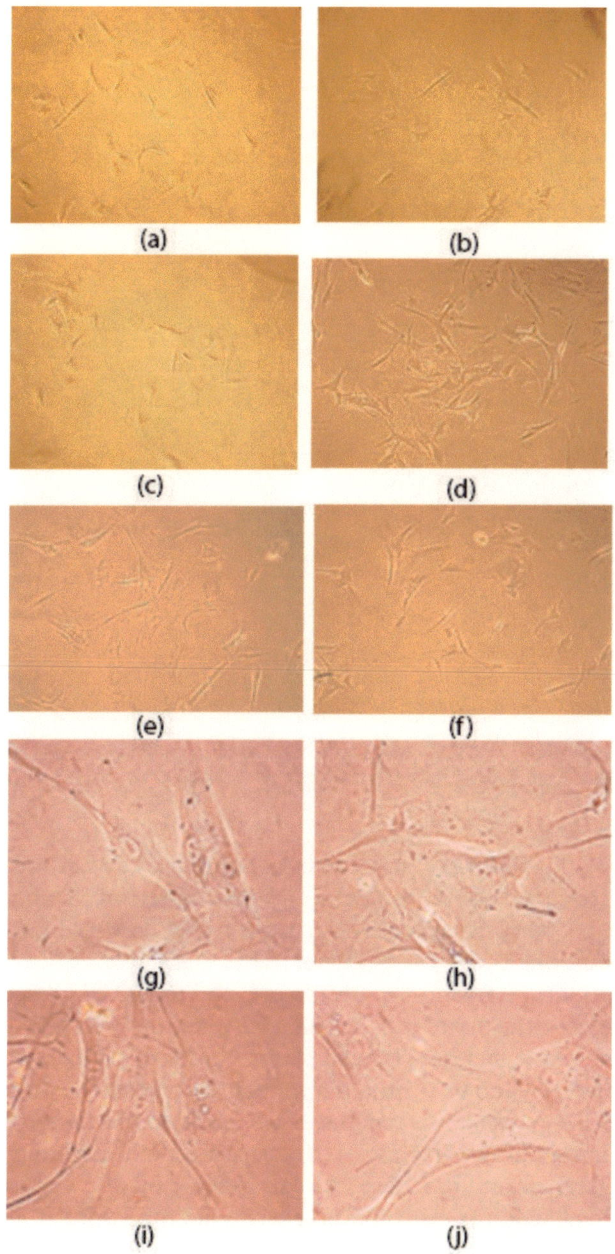

Figure 10.
Fibroblasts grown in DMEM (a, b, c, g, h) compared to fibroblasts grown in DMEM previously exposed to BTCM material for 24 h (d, e, f, i, j) (bright-field microscopy, 10× magnification, a–f, and 40× magnification, g–j).

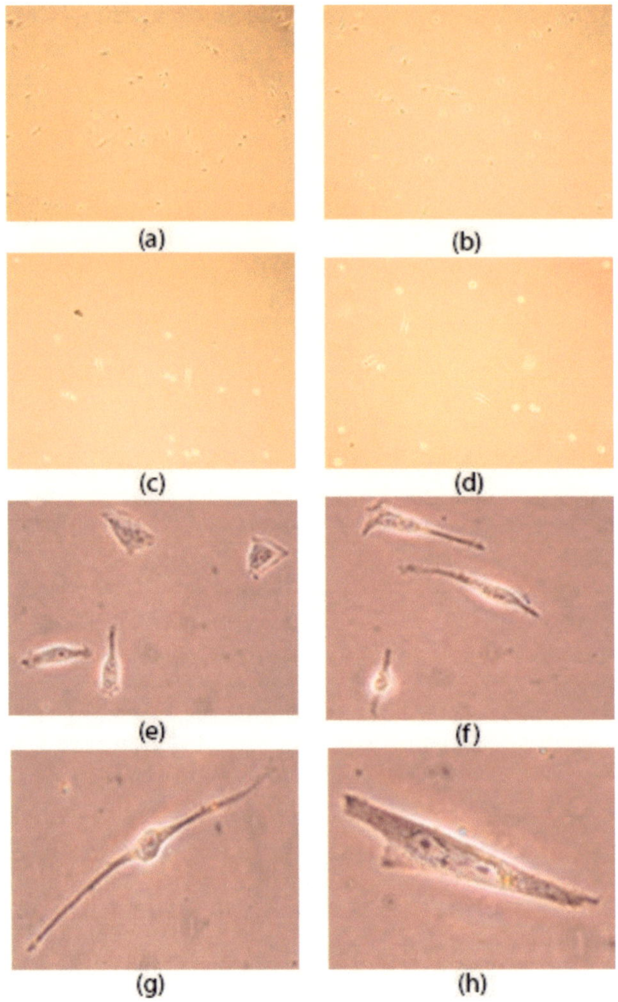

Figure 11.
SkMel23 cells grown in DMEM (a, b, e, f) compared to SKMel23 cells grown in DMEM previously exposed to BTCM material for 24 h (c, d, g, h) (bright-field microscopy 10× magnification, a–d and 40× magnification, e–h).

containing 100 × 10^4 SKMel23 cells in an 8 ml complete DMEM medium was added onto the sterilized BTCM material and previously preincubated in DMEM according to the protocol described above and further cultured for 24 h in complete DMEM medium.

After 24 h the culture medium was removed, and the BTCM material was washed three times with 8 ml of sterile PBS. The material was then moved using a sterile metal spatula to another six-well plate in order to evaluate only the cells adhered to the material and to exclude those that adhered to the plastic surface of the well. The BTCM material was incubated with 8 ml of sterile trypsin for 10 min, at 37°C with gentle shaking every 3 min to ensure a good detachment of cells. The supernatant was transferred to a 15 ml tube to which 6 ml of complete DMEM was added for trypsin neutralization and was centrifuged for 5 min, at 1500 rpm. The cell pellet was recovered at the bottom of the tube, and cells were counted after dilution 1/1 with trypan blue, which stains only the dead cells. From 100 × 10^4 SkMel23 cells seeded on BTCM material, a number of 8 × 10^4 cells were recovered after 24 h, which indicates that at least 8% of SkMel23 cells were able to adhere to BTCM material.

8. Conclusions

Materials based on BT or BST and collagen are candidates for medical applications in bone reconstruction and enhancement, suitable for 3D printing technologies that allow patient-specific shape, microstructure, and composition of the artificial bone. Artificial graft osteointegration at the interface with the natural bone will be facilitated by a printed porous structure that allows cellular infiltration, adherence, and growth. An example of ceramic-polymer hybrid material fabricated by 3D printing method was presented here. *For the first time*, 3D hybrid organic-inorganic materials based on barium titanate and collagen (BTC) and barium strontium titanate and collagen (BST-C), with potential applications as filler in bone tissue engineering, have been developed by integrating hydrothermal synthesis with additive manufacturing (extrusion-based 3D printing method). Morpho-structural characterization of 3D structures clearly showed multiple layers of fibers deposited at various angles in the 3D structure. Fiber thickness is around 500–600 μm in the case of BTCM sample. Both BTCM and BST-C samples are composed of spherical particles with crystallite size (estimated from X-ray diffraction patterns) of 14.1 nm (for BTCM) and 8.9 nm (for BST-C).

The 3D printed BTCM materials are physically stable and do not release toxic soluble compounds in cell culture medium. The BTCM material structure allows the adhesion of SkMel23 cells and possibly of other cell phenotypes as well. The cells recovered after being in contact with 3D printed BTCM materials are fully viable.

Mechanical properties of the 3D printed bone graft may be modulated at the nanometer scale by addition of collagen or other biopolymers into the printing paste, whereas at the microscale a composite structure could be completed by the infiltrating cells lying down on the collagen fibers. We propose some criteria to design bone materials that may share the remarkable toughness and self-repairing capabilities of the natural bone and the improved fracture resistance conferred by novel biopolymer-ceramic hybrid printing pastes. The 3D printing technology is thus suitable to address various bone pathologies, ranging from traumatic bone destruction to anomalous remodeling that occurs in osteoporosis. The results we presented here recommend the novel 3D structures as potentially biocompatible and support their use for further in vitro or animal model assays.

Acknowledgements

Financial support of National Core Programme project no. PN 18070101/2018 is gratefully acknowledged. The authors thank Eng. Raluca Elena Irimescu (IMNR) for the experimental work performed during STSM stage at Technion–Israel Institute of Technology in the frame of COST Action CA 15102, CRM-EXTREME. The authors also thank Ludmila Levin (Technion) for performing the SEM/EDX analysis and XRD analysis and Dudi Badler (Technion) for performing the optical profilometry measurement.

Conflict of interest

The authors declare no conflict of interest.

Author details

Roxana Mioara Piticescu[1], Laura Madalina Cursaru[1*], Gabriela Negroiu[2], Cristina Florentina Ciobota[1], Ciprian Neagoe[1] and Daniel Safranchik[3]

1 National R&D Institute for Non-Ferrous and Rare Metals—IMNR, Pantelimon, Romania

2 Institute of Biochemistry of the Romanian Academy—IBAR, Bucharest, Romania

3 Technion Research and Development Foundation, The Israel Institute of Metals, Technion Israel Institute of Technology, Haifa, Israel

*Address all correspondence to: mpopescu@imnr.ro

References

[1] Jazayeri HE, Rodriguez-Romero M, Razavi M, Tahriri M, Ganjawalla K, Rasoulianboroujeni M, et al. The cross-disciplinary emergence of 3D printed bioceramic scaffolds in orthopedic bioengineering. Ceramics International. 2018;**44**:1-9

[2] Tariverdian T, Behnamghader A, Milan PB, Barzegar-Bafrooei H, Mozafari M. 3D-printed barium strontium titanate-based piezoelectric scaffolds for bone tissue engineering. Ceramics International. 2019;**45**:14029-14038

[3] Jiao H, Zhao K, Bian T, Tang Y. Hydrothermal synthesis and properties characterization of barium titanate/hydroxyapatite spherical nanocomposite materials. Journal of Alloys and Compounds. 2017;**715**:73-82

[4] Ehterami A, Kazemi M, Nazari B, Saraeian P, Azami M. Fabrication and characterization of highly porous barium titanate based scaffold coated by Gel/HA nanocomposite with high piezoelectric coefficient for bone tissue engineering applications. Journal of the Mechanical Behavior of Biomedical Materials. 2018;**79**:195-202

[5] Tang Y, Wu C, Wu Z, Hu L, Zhang W, Zhao K. Fabrication and in vitro biological properties of piezoelectric bioceramics for bone regeneration. Scientific Reports. 2017;**43360**:1-12

[6] Anderson JC, Eriksson C. Piezoelectric properties of dry and wet bone. Nature. 1970;**227**:491-492

[7] Yasuda I. On the piezoelectric activity of bone. Journal of the Japanese Orthopedic Surgery Society. 1954;**28**:267

[8] Fukada E, Yasuda I. On the piezoelectric effect of bone. Journal of the Physical Society of Japan. 1957;**12**:1158-1162

[9] Bassett CA, Becker RO. Generation of electric potentials by bone in response to mechanical stress. Science. 1962;**28**:1063-1064

[10] Nakamura M, Hiratai R, Yamashita K. Bone mineral as an electrical energy reservoir. Journal of Biomedical Materials Research. Part A. 2012;**100**:1368-1374

[11] Bassett CA, Pawluk RJ, Becker RO. Effects of electric currents on bone in vivo. Nature. 1964;**204**:652-654

[12] McElhaney JH. The charge distribution on the human femur due to load. Journal of Bone and Joint Surgery. American Volume. 1967;**49**:1561-1571

[13] Park JB, Lake RS. Biomaterials: An Introduction. 2nd ed. New York: Plenum Press; 1992

[14] Wolff J The Law of Bone Remodelling. Berlin: Springer Verlag; 1986

[15] Zhang Y, Chen L, Zeng J, Zhou K, Zhang D. Aligned porous barium titanate/hydroxyapatite composites with high piezoelectric coefficients for bone tissue engineering. Materials Science and Engineering C. 2014;**39**:143-149

[16] Ribeiro C, Sencadas V, Correia DM, Lanceros-Méndez S. Piezoelectric polymers as biomaterials for tissue engineering applications. Colloid Surface B. 2015;**136**:46-55

[17] Rajabi AH, Jaffe M, Arinzeh TL. Piezoelectric materials for tissue regeneration: A review. Acta Biomaterialia. 2015;**24**:12-23

[18] Feng JQ, Yuan HP, Zhang XD. Promotion of osteogenesis by a

piezoelectric biological ceramic. Biomaterials. 1997;**18**:1531-1534

[19] Jones JR, Ehrenfried LM, Hench LL. Optimising bioactive glass scaffolds for bone tissue engineering. Biomaterials. 2006;**27**:964-973

[20] Khosla S, Westendorf JJ, Oursler MJ. Building bone to reverse osteoporosis and repair fractures. The Journal of Clinical Investigation. 2008;**118**:421-428

[21] Senatov FS, Niaza KV, Stepashkin AA, Kaloshkin SD. Low-cycle fatigue behavior of 3D-printed PLA-based porous scaffolds. Composites Part B: Engineering. 2016;**97**:193-200

[22] Zhong G, Vaezi M, Liu P, Pan L, Yang S. Characterization approach on the extrusion process of bioceramics for the 3D printing of bone tissue engineering scaffolds. Ceramics International. 2017;**43**:13860-13868

[23] Kim S, Ahn T, Han MH, Bae C, Oh DS. Wicking property of graft material enhanced bone regeneration in the ovariectomized rat model. Tissue Engineering and Regenerative Medicine. 2018;**15**(4):503-510

[24] Turnbull G, Clarke J, Picard F, Riches P, Jia L, Han F, et al. 3D bioactive composite scaffolds for bone tissue engineering. Bioactive Materials. 2018;**3**:278-314

[25] Schult M, Buckow E, Seitz H. Experimental studies on 3D printing of barium titanate ceramics for medical applications. Current Directions in Biomedical Engineering. 2016;**2**(1):95-99

[26] Gaytan SM, Cadena MA, Karim H, Delfin D, Lin Y, Espalin D, et al. Fabrication of barium titanate by binder jetting additive manufacturing technology. Ceramics International. 2015;**41**:6610-6619

[27] Griffith AA. The phenomena of rupture and flow in solids. Philosophical Transactions, Series A. 1921;**221**:163-198

[28] Irwin GR. Fracture dynamics. In: Fracturing of Metals. Cleveland, OH: American Society for Metals; 1948. pp. 147-166

[29] Orowan E. Fracture and strength of solids. Reports on Progress in Physics. 1949;**12**:185-232

[30] Roylance D. Introduction to fracture mechanics. In: 3.11 Mechanics of Materials. Massachusetts Institute of Technology: MIT OpenCourseWare; 2001. Available from: http://ocw.mit.edu/

[31] Chen PY, Lin AY, Lin YS, Seki Y, Stokes AG, Peyras J, et al. Structure and mechanical properties of selected biological materials. Journal of the Mechanical Behavior of Biomedical Materials. 2008;**1**:208-226

[32] Diaz-Rodriguez P, López-Álvarez M, Serra J, González P, Landín M. Current stage of marine ceramic grafts for 3D bone tissue regeneration. Marine Drugs. 2019;**17**(8):471. DOI: 10.3390/md17080471

[33] Linke WA, Hamdani N. Gigantic business: Titin properties and function through thick and thin. Circulation Research. 2014;**114**:1052-1068

[34] Improta S, Politou AS, Pastore A. Immunoglobulin-like modules from titin I-band: Extensible components of muscle elasticity. Structure. 1996;**4**:323-337

[35] Li H, Linke WA, Oberhauser AF, Carrion-Vazquez M, Kerkvliet JG, Lu H, et al. Reverse engineering of the giant muscle protein titin. Nature. 2002;**418**:998-1002

[36] Minajeva A, Kulke M, Fernandez JM, Linke WA. Unfolding of

titin domains explains the viscoelastic behavior of skeletal myofibrils. Biophysical Journal. 2001;**80**:1442-1451

[37] Bozec L, Horton M. Topography and mechanical properties of single molecules of type I collagen using atomic force microscopy. Biophysical Journal. 2005;**88**:4223-4231

[38] Linke WA, Kulke M, Li H, Fujita-Becker S, Neagoe C, Manstein DJ, et al. PEVK domain of titin: An entropic spring with actin-binding properties. Journal of Structural Biology. 2002;**137**:194-205

[39] Oroudjev E, Soares J, Arcdiacono S, Thompson JB, Fossey SA, Hansma HG. Segmented nanofibers of spider dragline silk: Atomic force microscopy and single-molecule force spectroscopy. Proceedings of the National Academy of Sciences of the United States of America. 2002;**99**:6460-6465

[40] Bozec L, van der Heijden G, Horton M. Collagen fibrils: Nanoscale ropes. Biophysical Journal. 2007;**92**:70-75

[41] Meyers MA, McKittrick J, Chen PY. Structural biological materials: Critical mechanics-materials connections. Science. 2013;**339**:773-779

[42] Wenger MPE, Bozec L, Horton M, Mesquida P. Mechanical properties of collagen fibrils. Biophysical Journal. 2007;**93**:1255-1263

[43] Piriou P, Ouenzerfi G, Migaud H, Renault E, Massi F, Serrault M. A numerical model to reproduce squeaking of ceramic-on-ceramic total hip arthroplasty. Influence of design and material. Orthopaedics & Traumatology, Surgery & Research. 2016;**102**:S229-S234